ABC of
Equality, Diversity and Inclusion in Healthcare

ABC of

Equality, Diversity and Inclusion in Healthcare

EDITED BY

Shehla Imtiaz-Umer

Equality, Diversity and Inclusion (EDI) Director, General Practice Task Force (GPTF) Derbyshire, UK
General Practitioner, Wilson Street Surgery, UK
GMC Associate, UK

John Frain

Division of Medical Sciences and Graduate Entry Medicine
University of Nottingham, UK

WILEY Blackwell

A catalogue record for this book is available from the Library of Congress

Paperback ISBN: 9781119875307; ePub ISBN: 9781119875321; ePDF ISBN: 9781119875314

Cover Design: Wiley
Cover Images: © The Good Brigade/Getty Images, ThisAbility Limited/Getty Images, kali9/Getty Images

Set in 9/12pt MinionPro by Integra Software Services Pvt. Ltd., Pondicherry, India
Printed and bound by CPI Group (UK) Ltd, Croydon, CR0 4YY

C9781119875307_260423

Contents

Preface

In their campaign 'Equality Matters', the British Medical Association (BMA) describes four key values. The first of these is:

"Equality matters because it's morally right"

The campaign goes on to describe further reasons that demonstrate why equality matters – maximising the potential of medical students and doctors, improving the performance and wellbeing of staff, and the benefits for patient care and healthcare systems. All of these are true, and there are substantial benefits for everyone, but it always comes around to the same starting point – equality and inclusion matter because they are morally right. They increase the chances of individuals and groups being able to fully be themselves, utilise their talents and fulfil their potential. Who could possibly not want that?

However, this is not the experience for many people and for many groups who find themselves marginalised not only by wider society but even by healthcare professionals and organisations within healthcare systems. There is ample evidence for this. Historical evidence but also evidence of attitudes and practices prevalent today which tell individual patients and staff 'You are not welcome here' or 'You do not belong here'. We cannot be bystanders to this and simply watch the effects on others – patients who lack the confidence to access healthcare, fearing how they will be received; colleagues, often more talented than ourselves, whose path is blocked by prejudice. Improving workplace diversity entails more than just implementing policies and procedures or increasing headcount or employment quotas; it also necessitates championing the unique aspects of every employee, regardless of their background. All of us need to reflect, examine our own attitudes and take steps to make ourselves and our teams in healthcare more inclusive to ensure patient safety is not compromised.

In authoring this book, we are responding to many enquiries and suggestions from our students and colleagues about how we can make our healthcare training more inclusive and representative. This has been an enriching experience both personally and professionally. We hope this book will be an educational resource to make a positive contribution to more inclusive curriculums and conversations about equality, diversity and inclusion (EDI) in healthcare. We also hope it will increase awareness of the substantial scientific and practical contributions made to healthcare by individuals from every single background.

We are grateful for the contribution of our authors, all of whom committed to their chapters during the COVID-19 pandemic, an event which has brought into much sharper focus so many of the themes we set out to explore in this book. Though we are based in the UK and the book reflects the perspective from the NHS, we are grateful for the contribution of colleagues in the United States. From our professional conversations, we believe the themes we have explored reflect concerns in many countries and health systems worldwide.

We hope the individual reader will find this book of interest and encouragement. Equality and inclusion matter because they are morally right. As so often with doing the right thing, we all benefit personally and professionally through improved wellbeing for staff and better outcomes for our patients.

Shehla Imtiaz-Umer
John Frain
October 2022

Contributors

Diana Akpeki LLB, LLM, PGCE

Final Year Graduate Entry Medical Student, University of Nottingham, Nottingham, UK

Mohammad Rizwan Ali BSc(Hons), MRes

PhD Fellow in Epidemiology, Department of Cardiovascular Sciences, College of Life Sciences, University of Leicester, Leicester, UK

Zunaira Dara BMBS, BSc(Hons), PGCert

Foundation Doctor, Greater Glasgow and Clyde, Scotland, UK

Anton Emmanuel MD, FRCP

Professor and Consultant Neurogastroenterologist, UCL, UCLH and NHNN; Lead of the Workforce Race Equality Standard and Interim Joint Director of Equality, Diversity and Inclusion, NHS England, University College London Hospitals, London, UK

Anna Frain MBChB, MRCGP, PGCert

GP Teaching Fellow, University of Nottingham, Nottingham, UK; Programme Director Derby Speciality Training Scheme for General Practice, Derby, UK; General Practitioner, Derwent Valley Medical Practice, Derby, UK

John Frain MB, ChB, MSc, FRCGP, DCH, DGM, DRCOG, PGDipCard, SFHEA

Clinical Associate Professor and Director of Clinical Skills, Division of Medical Sciences and Graduate Entry Medicine, University of Nottingham, Nottingham, UK

Lisa I. Iezzoni MD, MSc

Professor of Medicine, Health Policy Research Center, Mongan Institute, Massachusetts General Hospital; Department of Medicine, Harvard Medical School, Boston, USA

Shehla Imtiaz-Umer BSc(Hons), MSc, BMBS, MRCGP, DRCOG, DCH

Equality, Diversity, and Inclusion (EDI) Director General Practice Task Force (GPTF), Derbyshire; General Practitioner, Wilson Street Surgery, Derby, UK; GMC Associate, UK

Olivia King MSc, MBA, LLM

Senior Strategy and Policy Lead, NHS England, England

Diana Lautenberger MA

Director, Gender Equity Initiatives, Academic Affairs, Association of American Medical Colleges, Washington, DC, USA

Duncan McGregor BMBS, BSc

Core Trainee Doctor, North West School of Anaesthetics, Manchester, UK; LGBTQ+ Health Activist, Ex-Chair for GLADD – Association of LGBTQ+ Doctors and Dentists, London, UK

Habib Naqvi MBE, BSc, MSc, DHealthPsy

Director, NHS Race and Health Observatory, London, UK

Olivia O'Connell MBChB, MRCGP, DCH, DRCOG, DFSRH

GP Teaching Fellow, University of Nottingham, Nottingham, UK; General Practitioner, Osmaston Surgery, Derby, UK

Oluwaseun Oluwaranti MBCHB, FWACP, MRCPsych, EMBA

Higher Trainee in Forensic Psychiatry, Nottinghamshire Healthcare NHS Foundation Trust, Nottingham, UK

James Smith MBBS, MA, MSc, MSc

Honorary Research Fellow, Health in Humanitarian Crises Centre, London School of Hygiene and Tropical Medicine; Médecins Sans Frontières/Doctors Without Borders, England

Sylk Sotto-Santiago EdD, MBA, MPS

Associate Professor of Medicine, Vice-Chair for Diversity, Health Equity and Inclusion, Vice-Chair for Faculty Affairs and Professional Development, Indiana University School of Medicine, Indianapolis, IN, USA

CHAPTER 1

Why Inclusion Matters

Shehla Imtiaz-Umer[1] and John Frain[2]

[1] Equality, Diversity and Inclusion (EDI) Director, General Practice Task Force (GPTF) Derbyshire, UK; General Practitioner, UK; GMC Associate, UK

[2] General Practitioner and Clinical Associate Professor and Director of Clinical Skills, Division of Medical Sciences and Graduate Entry Medicine, University of Nottingham, Nottingham, UK

OVERVIEW

- Equality, diversity and inclusion in healthcare are issues of human dignity and patient safety.
- They are not gifts to be bestowed by the powerful and the privileged but basic rights which should be defended and developed by everyone.
- If equality and inclusion matter, they matter for everyone, and no one should be excluded.
- The evidence base for healthcare in marginalised groups needs to be robust and applied in training and service delivery.
- Equality is related to social justice and means fairness and opportunity for all.
- Increasing inclusion is an urgent priority in ensuring the future provision of health services.

Introduction

The NHS Constitution establishes the NHS's principles and values in England. It defines the rights patients, public and staff have, the pledges the NHS has made, and the responsibilities public, patients and staff have to one another for the NHS to operate fairly and effectively.

Behavioural science increasingly demonstrates the importance of healthcare culture in ensuring patient safety and staff wellbeing. A culture of rudeness within teams affects individual and team performance for both procedural and communication-based tasks [1]. A core value of the NHS is that 'Everyone counts'. Unfortunately, for many patients and staff, the lived reality of this value is very different. British Medical Association (BMA) reports on racism, LGBT+ staff and students, and sexism have highlighted poor experiences for groups whose characteristics are actually protected by law (see Further resources). Sometimes, it is literally a matter of life and death (Box 1.1).

Box 1.1 A matter of life and death.

In the NHS, 63% of healthcare workers who died due to COVID-19 were from Black, Asian and minority ethnic backgrounds, 64% of nurses who died were minority ethnic, and 95% of doctors who died were minority ethnic.

Studies by the BMA and reviews by the government revealed that minority doctors were twice as likely to say they felt pressured to work in risky environments without appropriate protective equipment.

In the UK, a survey of more than 16 000 doctors by the BMA (2022) found that 48% of the respondents reported buying personal protective equipment (PPE) for personal use or using donated PPE due to a lack of supplies at their workplaces. The survey also found that 65% of doctors said they felt 'partly or not at all protected'.

Source: BMA. How well protected was the medical profession from Covid-19? www.bma.org.uk/media/5644/bma-covid-review-1st-report-19-may-2022.pdf (accessed 25th October 2022)

Too often, we assume that values including freedom, democracy, equality, fraternity and liberty are fixed destinations at which humanity has arrived, never to look back. This is counter to the historical record and misunderstands that the need to develop and realise human rights for all is still evolving. Without continuing vigilance and commitment, freedom turns to slavery, democracy becomes a dictatorship and the inclusion of only some can lead to discrimination against others. We must all be alert in defending these values and, when necessary, active bystanders in preventing their elimination.

This book outlines historical and current priorities for equality, diversity and inclusion in healthcare. However, these are not exclusive to healthcare but values we should promote in wider society. This emphasises the healthcare professional's responsibility not only as a worker and clinician but also as a citizen [2].

What is meant by equality, diversity and inclusion?

Diversity in healthcare reflects the range of experiences and identities of all patients and staff. It is related to the range of differences in wider society; everyone should see themselves represented at all levels. These differences include:

- **demographic**, e.g. gender, disability, race, sexual orientation, social class, – and/or

- **cognitive**, i.e. people who have different ways of thinking, different viewpoints and different skill sets in a team or department.

Wherever there are patients from ethnic minorities, there should be staff and leadership from ethnic minorities, and the same for women, the LGBT+ community, the disabled and the elderly. A responsive health service recognises and understands these differences and how they relate to individual clinical needs, not cultural or other stereotypes.

Recognising differences and protecting diversity facilitate fairness, equality and equity. Patients should feel confident to access the care they are entitled to, be listened to and have their needs properly assessed, knowing they will receive treatment according to their individual needs. Staff should feel represented in their training (see Chapter 5) and have equity of opportunity to jobs and career progression, including positions of influence and leadership (see Chapter 3). Equality does not necessarily mean treating everyone the same. It does mean creating and facilitating attitudes where people feel they can be themselves and 'bring their whole self to any situation'. They should feel valued for both their individual talents and their contribution to the organisation.

Inclusion provides us with a sense of belonging. It is the extent to which staff or members of society believe they are valued by the community within which they live and work, receive fair and equitable treatment, and believe that they are encouraged to contribute to the effectiveness of the group. Being included allows us to release our energies by enabling us to be fully ourselves. Receiving respect increases our sense of self-esteem and gives us the confidence to speak up, to collaborate and, importantly, to raise concerns without fear of retribution. In inclusive organisations, there is [3]:

- more innovation
- greater employee engagement
- improved problem solving
- higher productivity
- more sustainable and fair decision making
- increased staff retention
- identification of development opportunities
- responsiveness in meeting the changing needs of service users
- a better experience for service users.

Equality and justice

Societies and organisations prioritising equality and inclusion aspire to fairness for all – of health access, pay, housing, employment opportunities and in the courts. Social justice ensures that individuals assume roles in society and receive their due. This requires removing barriers to social mobility and increasing the availability of safety nets for the vulnerable. The roots of social justice should be deep not only in the hearts and minds of all citizens but also in the institutions and bodies that regulate society. Governments and institutions should promote co-operation and social responsibility through policies on taxation, education, health and public services, employment rights, distribution of wealth and equity of opportunity (Figure 1.1).

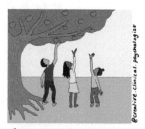

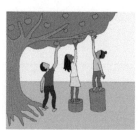

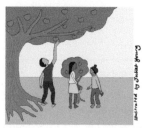

Figure 1.1 How equality relates to justice.
Source: © Dr Juliet Young, Clinical Psychologist, permission granted for use within this book.

The law

Given the historical and continuing injustices towards some communities, legal protection is required against discrimination (Box 1.2). In the UK, The Equality Act 2010 includes provisions that have direct implications for healthcare and serves as the legal framework for service delivery. It shapes our approach as both employers and key stakeholders in the system.

The Equality Act 2010 identifies nine protected characteristics:

- age
- disability
- gender reassignment
- marriage and civil partnership
- pregnancy and maternity
- race
- religion or belief
- sex
- sexual orientation.

The Human Rights Act 1998 protects people's human rights in the UK and enshrines the European Convention on Human Rights articles in British law. Protection is given against discrimination, harassment and victimisation (Box 1.2).

Box 1.2 **Definitions.**	
Direct discrimination	Someone is treated less favourably than someone else due to a protected characteristic, e.g. an employer refusing to recruit a woman over a man who is less qualified for the role is sex discrimination.

Indirect discrimination	When a rule or policy that applies to everyone puts a certain group at a disadvantage, e.g. a job advert for a ward sister says applicants must have spent 10 years working in the role. By doing this, the department could be discriminating indirectly based on age because younger people are excluded.
Discrimination by association	Direct discrimination towards an individual because they are associated with someone who has a protected characteristic, e.g. an employee is overlooked for overtime because they care for an elderly relative.
Discrimination by perception	Direct discrimination against someone because others perceive they have a protected characteristic even if they don't, e.g. refusing to work with someone with an Arabic name because you wrongly assume they're Muslim.
Harassment	Unwanted conduct that has the purpose or effect of violating a person's dignity or creating an intimidating, degrading, humiliating or offensive environment, e.g. a senior member of staff who makes sexual remarks or invitations to a younger member of staff.
Victimisation	Where someone is treated badly because they have made or supported a complaint under the Equality Act, e.g. a member of staff who has spoken up about an incident of religious discrimination and is then ostracised for having done so.

Why do equality, diversity and inclusion in healthcare matter?

Workforce

The NHS People Plan, published in July 2020, requires us to look after each other, foster a culture of compassion, inclusion and belonging, take action to grow our workforce, train our people and work together to deliver patient care. It outlines how the workforce can act with integrity, intelligence, empathy, openness and in the spirit of learning.

As COVID-19 has highlighted, we live in a society where patterns of discrimination and inequality dominate life chances, health status, education, housing, justice and employment and are influenced by our protected characteristics and birth class. Such factors significantly affect who is hired, how they advance, how they are treated and whether they continue their NHS career. Unfortunately, data on class and some other protected characteristics are lacking about recruitment, career progression and retention (Table 1.1) [4,5].

Critically, not ensuring equality, diversity and inclusivity within the workforce can impact patient care and become a safety issue. Data have repeatedly shown adverse patient outcomes due to discriminatory practices within the workforce (see Chapter 3).

Despite collecting national data over several years in secondary care to understand the disparity within the workforce, there has been little sustained positive shift in workplace experiences for racial

equality [6]. Discrimination experienced by NHS staff originates from both patients and colleagues. Whilst the focus on race discrimination has been challenged, the emphasis has been placed on this specific aspect as the dataset repeatedly demonstrates that discriminatory racial practices negatively impact patient outcomes [7].

While over 90% of patient consultations occur in primary care, there is no equivalent annual survey to understand the breadth and depth of discriminatory practices in general practice. Local teams have taken the initiative to understand the issues facing their workplaces. Every GP team undertaking a workforce survey has identified racial, ethnic or religious discrimination (see Chapters 2 and 3) (Box 1.3).

Box 1.3 Experiences of discrimination in non-hospital services in England [8,9].

The WRES (Table 1.1) does not cover primary care personnel or wider medical and dental personnel, even though over 60% of general practitioners (GPs) are people from a Black or ethnic minority background.

The first comprehensive primary care workforce survey was undertaken in London by NHS England and Health Education England in 2022, after smaller, local surveys were completed in areas including Humberside, Derbyshire and Leeds.

'Experiences of racial discrimination and harassment in London Primary Care' data showed that race was the most common characteristic associated with harassment and discrimination, above gender, age, religion and disability. Of those surveyed for the study:

- 1 in 3 reported racial discrimination or harassment from patients in the past 12 months (30%) and about 1 in 5 from staff they worked with (18%)
- People from Black and Asian heritage groups were most likely to say they had experienced racial discrimination or harassment from patients and colleagues.

'Unconscious bias is sewn into the fabric of the NHS. Very junior, inexperienced White colleagues were invited to senior positions ... Relevant experience with additional qualifications is discarded if you are non-White ... Ethnic minorities are there to do the coal face work whilst White colleagues get promoted to managerial and strategic roles.'

(Quote from GP participant in the study)

Source: Experiences of Racial Discrimination and Harassment in London Primary Care, 2022 www.hee.nhs.uk/sites/default/files/documents/Pan-LondonDiscrimination%26RacismPrimaryCareSurvey_Final.pdf (accessed 25th October 2022)

Improving workplace diversity entails more than just implementing policies and procedures or increasing headcount or employment quotas; it also necessitates championing the unique aspects of every employee, regardless of their background, and actively calling out discrimination (see Chapter 12).

This includes examining how we recruit, retain and develop our workforce and how we support their wellbeing. It requires an assessment of how representative our leadership teams are and whether our workforce data reveal any disparities in representation based on any of the nine protected characteristics outlined in The Equality Act 2010.

Table 1.1 Summary of Workforce Race Equality Standards (WRES) from 2016 to 2020.

	2016	2017	2018	2019	2020
Relative likelihood of White applicants being appointed from shortlisting across all posts compared to BME applicants[1]	1.57	1.6	1.45	1.46	1.61
Relative likelihood of BME staff entering the formal disciplinary process compared to White staff[2]	1.56	1.37	1.24	1.22	1.16
Percentage of staff experiencing harassment, bullying or abuse from patients, relatives or the public in last 12 months. White staff shown in brackets[3]	28.4 (27.5)	28.5 (27.7)	29.7 (27.8)	30.3 (27.9)	28.9 (25.9)
Percentage of staff who personally experienced discrimination at work from a manager, team leader or other colleagues. White staff shown in brackets	14.0 (6.1)	14.5 (6.1)	15.0 (6.6)	14.5 (6.0)	16.7 (6.2)
Percentage of BME staff believing that trust provides equal opportunities for career progression or promotion. White staff shown in brackets[4]	73.2 (87.8)	71.9 (86.8)	69.9 (86.3)	71.2 (86.9)	69.2 (87.3)

This table shows the various trends in data which reflect challenges in discrimination faced by staff from colleagues as well as members of the public.
[1]White applicants were significantly more likely than BME applicants to be appointed from shortlisting.
[2]In 50% of NHS trusts BME staff were more than 1.25 times more likely than White staff to enter the formal disciplinary process. There has been a reduction in the likelihood to be referred for formal disciplinary processes.
[3]Since 2015, a higher percentage of BME employees has been harassed, bullied or abused by patients, family or the general public than White employees. In 2020, it is still higher for BME staff (28.9% compared to White staff – 25.9%) The recent decline could be due to the impact of the COVID-19 pandemic, which reduced the amount of face-to-face contact between patients or service users and those providing NHS care.
[4]This is now at its lowest point since 2015.
Source: www.england.nhs.uk/wp-content/uploads/2022/04/Workforce-Race-Equality-Standard-report-2021-.pdf (accessed 24th October 2022)

When staff are not welcomed, their differences are not valued and there is no safe place for them to raise concerns or admit mistakes, patient care suffers. However, demographic diversity supported by inclusion can significantly improve creativity, innovation and productivity.

Patients

The NHS seeks to reduce health inequalities and discrimination against patients and staff. People become ill as a result of discrimination. For over two decades, we have known that aside from socioeconomic effects, both experiences of racial harassment and perceptions of racial discrimination make an independent contribution to health [7]. For example, those who are verbally harassed have a 50% greater chance of reporting fair or poor health than those who have not been harassed [7] (see Chapter 2). Racism is a recognised social determinant of health and contributes to ethnic health disparities.

Race discrimination is associated with a range of adverse outcomes, including coronary heart disease, worse maternal and neonatal outcomes, high blood pressure, lower birth weight, cognitive impairment and mortality. Additionally, in witnessed out-of-hospital cardiac arrest, Black and Hispanic persons are less likely than White persons to receive potentially lifesaving bystander CPR (see Further Resources). Discrimination, like other stressors, can have an impact on health through both actual exposure and the threat of exposure to discriminatory practices. Feeling excluded increases the risk of depression and psychological alienation, as well as poor cognitive functioning, impaired motivation and poor physical health (see Chapters 6, 7 and 10). The desire to belong is a strong human motivation.

By extrapolating the experiences of racial discrimination to other protected characteristics, we can begin to understand the cumulative effect of these discriminatory practices on the health outcomes of many marginalised members of our society, including women and the LGBTQ+ community. These groups are ideologically assigned a different value, which leads to disparities in power, resources and opportunities. This intersectional identity can lead to the observed differential in privilege and power happening at both structural and individual levels (see Chapter 11).

Ageism

A protected characteristic shared by all is age. We are all mortal yet even here, there is inequality of experience. The healthcare impacts of ageing include effects on: [10]

- healthcare seeking behaviour
- diagnosis and treatment recommendations
- internalised beliefs about ageing producing weakness and dependence on others
- attitudes and reduced respect towards older patients
- dismissing patients' symptoms as 'just old age'.

This can affect women disproportionately, and they may be refused more aggressive treatments due to perceived increased frailties [10]. Ageism may intersect with other marginalised identities, including gender, race and sexual orientation. Black patients with dementia were more than twice as likely to contract and die from COVID-19 than White patients [11]. Ageism affects the LGBT+ community, who report difficulties establishing social spaces and accessing healthcare, housing, social service and legal assistance. This affects those more who have felt less able to disclose their sexuality at a younger age [12].

Religious discrimination

We live in a society with an ever-expanding and diverse mix of religions and beliefs, which NHS organisations must consider when developing both public services and employment policies. Even within established religions, there are different branches and regional and sectional variants with different interpretations, rituals, moral guidelines, traditions and laws. Personal compliance can range from nominal to strict adherence. Furthermore, many people have strong feelings about not having a personal religious belief.

Additionally, research has revealed differences in the health and wellbeing of various religious communities, which provides an opportunity to target services. For example, the British Muslim community has the worst reported health, followed by the Sikh population. Females are more likely to report illness in both groups, as well as Hindus, whereas Christians and Jews have only a minor gender difference. It should be noted that this is not always a case of cause and effect but is more likely to be influenced by other factors such as the social determinants of health (see Chapter 4) [13].

The pandemic also highlighted the importance of providing faith-specific guidance in a culturally and linguistically specific context [14]. The success of this work has highlighted the importance of understanding the challenges faced by faith groups in accessing healthcare (Box 1.4).

Box 1.4 **Faith-specific health inequalities review.**

Low immunisations, high COVID-19 rates, and increased breast cancer risks – some of several health inequalities disproportionally found amongst Jewish communities in England. The NHS Race Health Observatory is undertaking a review to better understand the barriers to healthcare faced specifically by the Jewish community. The wide-ranging review will aim to include several factors, including the impact of communication in the following areas:
- Hospital food for patients.
- Difficulties with booking appointments, including on the sabbath and during religious festivals.
- Poor experience due to staff educational/cultural incompetency.
- Experience and impact of antisemitism from staff, patients or members of the public.
- End-of-life care, including care of the bereaved.
- Challenges in making use of trusted sources of health information from within the community.

Source: NHS Race Health Observatory. 2022. www.nhsrho.org/news/new-review-to-examine-health-inequalities-in-jewish-communities (accessed 25th October 2022)

The impact of religious discrimination must also be considered in the context of the workforce. Religious beliefs can profoundly affect how employees do their jobs. Because so few studies collect data on people's faith, research on the intersection of religion and the workplace is scarce.

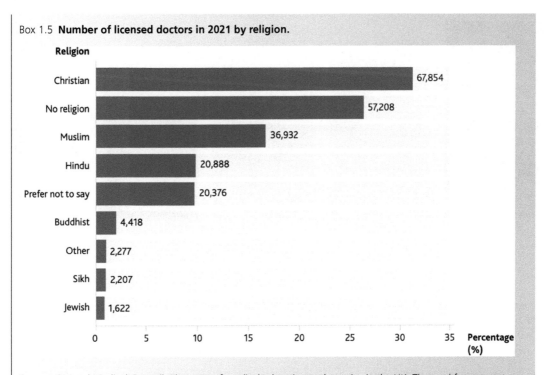

Box 1.5 **Number of licensed doctors in 2021 by religion.**

Religion	Number
Christian	67,854
No religion	57,208
Muslim	36,932
Hindu	20,888
Prefer not to say	20,376
Buddhist	4,418
Other	2,277
Sikh	2,207
Jewish	1,622

Percentage (%)

Source: General Medical Council. The state of medical education and practice in the UK: The workforce report 2022. www.gmc-uk.org/-/media/documents/workforce-report-2022---full-report_pdf-94540077.pdf (accessed 24th October 2022).

Since 2016, all doctors who register with the General Medical Council (GMC) for the first time are asked to provide information about their sexual orientation, religion, or belief, and whether they are disabled (Box 1.5) [15].

The lack of any significant empirical research in this area indicates a critical gap in our understanding of workplace religious discrimination. A workforce analysis by the King's Fund showed that people from all religions report experiencing discrimination based on their faith. Still, reporting is by far the highest among Muslims (Box 1.6) [16]. Staff belonging to any faith group continue to report discrimination and harassment (BMA, 2022 – see Further reading).

Specific workplace policies can result in reduced access to career opportunities due to religiously discordant practices such as 'bare below the elbow' and a ban on wearing hijab in theatres. The lack of whole-system engagement in overcoming these barriers has resulted in some healthcare-related faith groups, such as the British Islamic Medical Association, having to innovate and provide religious-specific solutions to the issues faced by their colleagues [17]. Muslim doctors report discrimination within dress code policies, and the Prevent policy fostered an institutional culture of fear and mistrust of Muslim colleagues. Notwithstanding the imperative of patient safety and infection control, solutions still need to be negotiated respectfully and be inclusive of everyone. The experience of Muslims is not unique – the King's Fund report [16] highlighted that Hindu colleagues also experience higher rates of discrimination based on their ethnic background, demonstrating the impact of having intersectional identities.

Religion should be considered in the drive for equality and diversity to ensure that healthcare systems are truly inclusive and compassionate for both staff and patients.

Improving the evidence base

Being fully inclusive is not just about having visual changes. These changes are relatively straightforward but unless there is better inclusion of content and evidence in policy, education and training reflected in the attitudes of all patients and staff, visual change only risks being perceived as tokenism. Whilst inclusive and visible diverse leadership is critical, there also need to be a cultural change and system shifts to ensure that people of all backgrounds can progress through their chosen careers. It is only by being authentic and compassionate that there will be an improvement in not only health but also social equity.

The research base of equality, diversity and inclusion needs urgent improvement. The misconceptions about ethnicity and disease (see Chapter 4), women's health (see Chapter 6), LGBT+ healthcare (see Chapter 7) and mental health (Chapter 10) need to be corrected (Boxes 1.7, 1.8, and 1.9). These include issues around:

Box 1.6 **Religious discrimination in the NHS.**

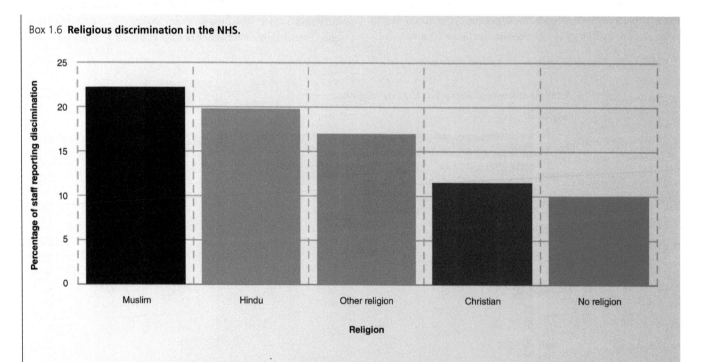

Overall discrimination is reported most by Muslim (22.2%) and Hindu (19.4%) staff, compared with staff of no religion (10.0%). Reported discrimination on the basis of religion is highest by far among Muslims (8%), followed by those of other religions (all religions not including Christians, Muslims and Hindus 1.9%), Hindus (1.3%), Christians (0.4%) and staff of no religion (0.2%).

Muslims and Hindus also report a far higher rate of discrimination on the basis of ethnic background.

Source: West, M., Dawson, J. and Kaur, M. (2015) Making the difference. Diversity and inclusion in the NHS. The King's Fund. www.kingsfund.org.uk/sites/default/files/field/field_publication_file/Making-the-difference-summary-Kings-Fund-Dec-2015.pdf (accessed 24th October 2022).

- the social determinants of health
- presentation of symptoms in women
- the experience of accessing healthcare by LGBT+ patients
- mental health in patients and staff with protected characteristics.

Box 1.7 **Impact of colonialism.**

The disease profile for non-communicable diseases, particularly type 2 diabetes (T2D), is on the rise in South Asian countries [18], with disparities between people of European ancestry compared to South Asian ancestry being particularly stark [19]. The differences in the prevalence of T2D between Europeans and South Asians have been postulated to be linked to lean free mass (muscle and organ mass), with ethnic-specific differences consistently reporting lower lean mass for South Asians compared to other ethnicities [20,21].

These differences in lean body mass could be a key signal for why Asians are more likely to develop T2D compared to their European counterpart. An adaptation to the many famines that were experienced in the nineteenth and twentieth centuries, which led to increased mortality, may have contributed to the selection pressures on genes [22]. This meant that these genes allowed the excess storage of calories, allowing South Asians to survive periods of famine adequately, yet increased body weight compared to their height. This postulated adaptation shows that global weather patterns and, more recently, racist and colonial policies may have led to generational negative health consequences for South Asians for developing T2D.

Box 1.8 **Race correction in obstetric algorithms.**

An example in obstetrics is the vaginal birth after caesarean (VBAC) score. This algorithm identifies that non-White mothers have a lower likelihood of success than White mothers. However, ethnicity is not incorporated into the algorithm, and non-White women have higher caesarean section rates than White women. Given the increased morbidity associated with caesarean section, using a score that underestimates successful birth outcomes for ethnic minority mothers is striking, given the up to fivefold increase in mortality seen in non-White mothers.

Source: Vyas, D.A., Eisenstein, L.G. and Jones, D.S. (2020) Hidden in plain sight – reconsidering the use of race correction in clinical algorithms. *New England Journal of Medicine*, **383**(9), 874–882.

Box 1.9 **Regulatory inequalities due to patient demographics.**

'We have a much younger population compared to … nationally, and […] the majority of these patients have English as a second language. Our CCG as a whole has the second highest proportion nationally of [Black and Ethnic Minority] patients (I think). Our population is much more deprived with some of the highest incidences of [Serious Mental Illness], with double the national prevalence of type 2 diabetes. Many of our newly registered patients have only recently arrived in the UK, mainly from Romania, Afghanistan, Iraq and Iran. These patients have massively complex needs – either

---

due to not having access to healthcare for many years, mental and physical health issues due to their traumatic experiences, poverty and different health beliefs due to cultural factors.' (Quote from GP, London, in Care Quality Commission 2021 report on minority-led general practice services)

Source: Care Quality Commission (2022) Ethnic minority-led GP practices: impact and experience of CQC regulation. www.cqc.org.uk/publications/themed-work/ethnic-minority-led-gp-practices-impact-experience-cqc-regulation (accessed 25th October 2022)

What does the future hold?

There has to be political will and recognition of ongoing issues, but we must move from reports and analysis to positive action. One recent development is the NHS commitment to investigating racial inequalities for the first time [23]. Unfortunately, at the time of writing, the Secretary of State for Health had shelved plans to publish a White Paper on the stark health inequalities exposed by the COVID-19 pandemic.

Both the UK's GMC and BMA have incorporated into their core documentation specific guidance for professionals and patients on the need for better care for all patients. They are also providing leadership in ensuring that the needs of marginalised groups such as LGBT+ and migrants are better addressed (Box 1.10).

Box 1.10 **General Medical Council – LGBT patient guide.**

Your rights as lesbian, gay, bi and trans patients

All patients must be able to trust doctors with their lives and health. They should all be treated with dignity and respect, regardless of their sexual orientation or gender identity.

This guide explains the standards that lesbian, gay, bi and trans (LGBT) patients should expect from their doctor; what we're doing to support LGBT patients; and information about organisations that provide advice or advocacy services.

Source: General Medical Council. LGBT patient guide. www.gmc-uk.org/ethical-guidance/patient-guides-and-materials/lgbt-patient-guide (accessed 25th October 2022)

Discriminatory incidents occur daily, and there needs to be more understanding about how one can address these instances. There are steps we can take within our spheres of influence, even if that is a single interpersonal interaction; everyone has the potential to change the outcome of a possible discriminatory experience. Chapter 12 outlines the importance of being an ally and how to be an active bystander, which we hope our readers will be able to implement immediately (Box 1.11).

Box 1.11 **I saw … but I did not speak out.**

I saw a Black patient being refused adequate pain relief
And I did not speak out

Because I am not Black
I saw a Gay colleague being denied a job opportunity
And I did not speak out
Because I am not Gay
I saw a junior female colleague being harassed
And I did not speak out
Because I am not a woman
I saw a disabled patient who needed workplace adaptations
And I did not speak out
Because I am not disabled
I saw a Transgender patient being ridiculed
And I did not speak out
Because I am not Transgender
I saw someone unable to keep their religious observance
And I did not speak out
Because I am not religious
I saw a talented Asian nurse denied a leadership position
And I did not speak out
Because I am neither Asian nor a nurse
I saw an elderly man being spoken to like a child
And I did not speak out
Because I am not elderly
Then I needed someone
To speak up for me
But I had not enabled anyone to help me

Source: Adapted from Pastor Martin Niemoller, 'First they came' (1946)

However, there are changes we can make within our organisations and educational institutions. Chapter 13 provides valuable guidance on how we can better train future colleagues.

Content of this work

It is outside the scope of this book to address each protected characteristic in detail. We have introduced key concepts and historical context to the issues identified as perpetuating discriminatory experiences within the workforce but also, more worryingly, against our patients. This is not to diminish the experiences of other protected characteristics; we have attempted to ensure all are mentioned.

Terminology is important and particular terms, including proper pronunciation of names, is valuable in signalling respect to a person. We recognise there is ongoing debate regarding the use of 'BAME', 'ethnic minority', LGBT+ and terms of reference to communities containing various cultures. We have not requested our authors to use particular terms but let them use the terminology with which they are most comfortable.

Conclusion

Our ability to provide comprehensive healthcare is currently in jeopardy. The most important resource – the people in it – is being squandered, with problems in both recruitment and retention. Addressing equality, diversity and inclusion is vital in remedying this. How urgent is this? In the extreme. How soon should we start? Yesterday

would have been ideal; tomorrow will be too late. Today is the time. These problems are made by human beings, so we can solve them by being bigger than who we are or believe ourselves to be.

'Change will not come if we wait for some other person or some other time. We are the ones we've been waiting for. We are the change we seek.' (Barack Obama)

Further reading/resources

Civility Saves Lives. www.civilitysaveslives.com (accessed 26th October 2022)

BMA (2016) The experience of lesbian, gay and bisexual doctors in the NHS. British Medical Association. www.bma.org.uk/media/4225/bma_experience-of-lgb-doctors-and-medical-students-in-nhs-2016.pdf (accessed 26th October 2022)

BMA (2022) Racism in medicine. British Medical Association. www.bma.org.uk/media/5746/bma-racism-in-medicine-survey-report-15-june-2022.pdf (accessed 26th October 2022)

BMA (2021) Sexism in medicine. British Medical Association. www.bma.org.uk/media/4487/sexism-in-medicine-bma-report.pdf (accessed 26th October 2022)

Department of Health and Social Security (1980) *Inequalities in Health: Report of a Research Working Group*. London: Department of Health and Social Security.

Garcia, R.A., Spertus, J., Girotra, S., et al (2022). Racial and ethnic differences in bystander CPR for witnessed cardiac arrest. *New England Journal of Medicine*, **387** (17), https://www.nejm.org/doi/full/10.1056/NEJMoa2200798 (accessed 27th October 2022)

NHS East of England (2021) No more tick boxes: a review on the evidence on how to make recruitment and career progression fairer. www.england.nhs.uk/east-of-england/wp-content/uploads/sites/47/2021/10/NHSE-Recruitment-Research-Document-FINAL-2.2.pdf (accessed 26th October 2022)

NHS People Plan 2020–21. www.england.nhs.uk/ournhspeople (accessed 26th October 2022)

Strategic Review of Health Inequalities in England post-2010 (2010) *Fair Society, Healthier Lives: The Marmot Review*. www.instituteofhealthequity.org/resources-reports/fair-society-healthy-lives-the-marmot-review/fair-society-healthy-lives-full-report-pdf.pdf (accessed 27th October 2022)

West, M., Dawson, J. and Kaur, M. (2015) Making the difference. Diversity and inclusion in the NHS. www.kingsfund.org.uk/sites/default/files/field/field_publication_file/Making-the-difference-summary-Kings-Fund-Dec-2015.pdf (accessed 26th October 2022)

References

1 Riskin, A., Erez, A., Foulk, T.A. et al. (2015) The impact of rudeness on medical team performance: a randomized trial. *Pediatrics*, **136** (3), 487–495.

2 Chandratilake, M., McAleer, S., Gibson, J., and Roff, S. (2010) Medical professionalism: what does the public think? *Clinical Medicine*, **10**, 364–369.

3 Page, S.E. (2017) *The Diversity Bonus: How Great Teams Pay Off in the Knowledge Economy*. Princeton University Press.

4 Health Foundation Health equity in England: the Marmot review 10 years on. www.health.org.uk/publications/reports/the-marmot-review-10-years-on?gclid=Cj0KCQjwsLWDBhCmARIsAPSL3_3yEX

Xvf-IY6NivspQad6b9ubn3t_a0-k0vuXCH3jufFMlZ2ToyErIaAvM2 EALw_wcB (accessed 25th October 2022)

5 Health Foundation Build back fairer: the Covid-19 Marmot review. www. health.org.uk/publications/build-back-fairer-the-covid-19-marmot-review (accessed 25th October 2022)

6 NHS England NHS workforce race equality standard. www.england.nhs. uk/about/equality/equality-hub/workforce-equality-data-standards/ equality-standard (accessed 25th October 2022)

7 Karlsen, S. and Nazroo, J. (2002). Agency and structure: the impact of ethnic identity and racism on the health of ethnic minority people. *Sociology of Health and Illness*, **24** (1), 1–20.

8 NHS England and NHS Improvement Experiences of racial discrimination and harassment in London primary care. (2022). www.hee.nhs.uk/sites/ default/files/documents/Pan-LondonDiscrimination%26RacismPrimary CareSurvey_Final.pdf (accessed 25th October 2022)

9 Humberside LMCs (2021) Racism and Discrimination – the experience of primary care professionals in the Humberside region. https://s3.eu-west-2.amazonaws.com/files.fourteenfish.com/websitefiles/ 26/13925/Racism%20survey%20report_final_amended_10052021.pdf? X-Amz-Expires=600&X-Amz-Algorithm=AWS4-HMAC-SHA256&X-Amz-Credential=AKIAU2VMDQYPZ55JOYGD/20221024/eu-west-2/ s3/aws4_request&X-Amz-Date=20221024T202019Z&X-Amz-Signed Headers=host&X-Amz-Signature=4c90cbe1424f7861184f8b08685a4a87 c5a9a79521c5b83a5b2cb2f5af235619 (accessed 25th October 2022).

10 Chrisler, J.C., Barney, A. and Palatino, B. (2016) Ageism can be hazardous to women's health: ageism, sexism, and stereotypes of older women in the healthcare system. *Journal of Social Issues*, **72** (1), 86–104.

11 Wang, Q., Davis, P.B., Gurney, M.E. and Xu, R. (2021) COVID-19 and dementia: analyses of risk, disparity, and outcomes from electronic health records in the US. *Alzheimers and Dementia*, **17** (8), 1297–1306.

12 Boggs, J., Portz, J.D., Wright, L. et al. (2014) D3-4: the intersection of ageism and heterosexism: LGBT older adults' perspectives on aging-in-place. *Clinical Medicine and Research*, **12** (1–2), 101.

13 Department of Health. Religion or belief. A practical guide for the NHS. www.clatterbridgecc.nhs.uk/application/files/7214/3445/0178/ ReligionorbeliefApracticalguidefortheNHS.pdf (accessed 27th October 2022)

14 Swihart, D.L., Yarrarapu, S.N.S. and Martin, R.L. (2022) Cultural religious competence in clinical practice. www.ncbi.nlm.nih.gov/books/NBK493216

15 General Medical Council. The state of medical education and practice in the UK: the workforce report 2022. www.gmc-uk.org/about/what-we-do-and-why/data-and-research/the-state-of-medical-education-and-practice-in-the-uk/workforce-report-2022 (accessed 25th October 2022)

16 West, M., Dawson, J. and Kaur, M. (2015) Making the difference. Diversity and inclusion in the NHS. www.kingsfund.org.uk/sites/default/files/field/ field_publication_file/Making-the-difference-summary-Kings-Fund-Dec-2015.pdf (accessed 25th October 2022)

17 Malik, A., Qureshi, H., Abdul-Razakq, H. et al. (2019) '*I decided not to go into surgery due to dress code*': a cross-sectional study within the UK investigating experiences of female Muslim medical health professionals on bare below the elbows (BBE) policy and wearing headscarves (hijabs) in theatre. *BMJ Open*, **9**, e019954.

18 Jayawardena, R. et al. (2012) Prevalence and trends of the diabetes epidemic in South Asia: a systematic review and meta-analysis. *BMC Public Health*, **12**: 380.

19 Gujral, U.P., Pradeepa, R., Weber, M.B. et al. (2013) Type 2 diabetes in South Asians: similarities and differences with white Caucasian and other populations. *Annals of the New York Academy of Sciences*, **1281**, 51–63.

20 Rush, E.C., Freitas, I. and Plank, L.D. (2009) Body size, body composition and fat distribution: comparative analysis of European, Maori, Pacific Island and Asian Indian adults. *British Journal of Nutrition*, **102**, 632–641.

21 Hull, H.R. et al. (2011) Fat-free mass index: changes and race/ ethnic differences in adulthood. *International Journal of Obesity*, **35**, 121–127.

22 Pomeroy, E., Mushrif-Tripathy, V., Cole, T.J. et al. (2011) Ancient origins of low lean mass among South Asians and implications for modern type 2 diabetes susceptibility. *Scientific Reports*, **9**, 10515.

23 NHS Race & Health Observatory. Public Digital announced to lead Observatory's Sickle Cell Disease digital discovery project. www. nhsrho.org/news/public-digital-announced-to-lead-observatorys-sickle-cell-disease-digital-discovery-project (accessed 25th October 2022)

CHAPTER 2

The Impact of Bias in Healthcare

Habib Naqvi

Director, NHS Race and Health Observatory, UK

OVERVIEW

- Bias can take different forms and negatively impact people's mental and physical health.
- Bias built into healthcare policies and processes can place patients at risk and harm them.
- Debiasing medical research and policy can benefit everyone.
- It is not always easy to unlearn biases, but it is important to do so for the betterment of society.
- Common, helpful actions can be taken to identify and help unlearn biases – such as learning about other cultures, ethnicities and identities.

Definitions

Often, we recognise bias as a natural inclination for or against an idea, object, group or individual. However, it is also learnt and is highly dependent on variables such as a person's religious beliefs, race, ethnicity, sex and educational background. At the individual level, bias can negatively affect someone's health and personal and professional relationships; at a societal level, it can lead to unfair treatment of a group or community. Examples of this in history include apartheid and slavery (Box 2.1).

Box 2.1 **Examples of social justice and bias issues facing the world.**

Slavery – you would think that slavery was a non-issue in current culture. However, it is still a social injustice issue found around the world.

Racial segregation – a famous historical example was the segregation of Black Americans in the US via Jim Crow laws. Another example of segregation was apartheid in South Africa.

Ageism – the elderly are discriminated against, creating negative stereotypes of the elderly as being weak, feeble or unable to change. A few examples include being denied work or being seen as a societal burden.

Pay gap – when it comes to pay in the workplace, there is a noticeable differentiation by, for example, gender and ethnicity.

LGBTQ+ – individuals of the Lesbian, Gay, Bisexual, Transsexual and Queer (LGBTQ) community face several forms of social injustice and oppression. For example, same-sex marriages are outlawed in some states in the USA and countries.

Poverty – when you think of poverty, you might think of having little food or living in a homeless shelter. However, the sad truth is that many individuals do not have access to food, clean water, schooling, healthcare or even sanitation.

Indeed, some biases can be positive and helpful, like choosing to eat foods that are considered healthy or making a conscious decision not to buy products from a company that has knowingly caused harm to others. However, biases are often based on stereotypes rather than on any actual evidence base associated with an individual or circumstance. Whether positive or negative, such cognitive shortcuts can result in prejudgements that can lead to rash decision making or discriminatory practices.

The Equality Act 2010 applies to everyone in Britain. It aims to protect people from discrimination, harassment and victimisation based on age, disability, gender reassignment, marriage and civil partnership, pregnancy and maternity, race, religion or belief, sex and sexual orientation.

Thus, what is the relationship between bias and discrimination? Discrimination is the unjust treatment of people based on the groups or classes they belong to. It is an action that stems from an attitudinal bias: when we misunderstand someone different from us, we treat them differently. This misunderstanding can be caused by implicit or explicit bias.

Understanding bias

Bias arises from our tendency to sort people into groups while also paying attention to what kinds of people are most likely to have power and resources in a society. Noticing that specific kinds of characteristics, for example, age, race and gender, are associated with having more or less

---

ABC of Equality, Diversity and Inclusion in Healthcare, First Edition. Edited by Shehla Imtiaz-Umer and John Frain.
© 2023 John Wiley & Sons Ltd. Published 2023 by John Wiley & Sons Ltd.

status, power, resources or respect from others can lead to judgements about people or groups. This way of attaching social value to particular characteristics is what leads to bias: a disproportionate preference for (or, on the other hand, an aversion to) an idea or a group of people, usually in a way that is closed-minded or unfair. This, in turn, can create discriminatory behaviours, practices and institutional policies.

Implicit bias

Implicit bias is often viewed as an unconscious or immediate thought process that may go directly against our conscious beliefs. Bias comes from natural tendencies coupled with what we *learn* and *observe*, starting at a very young age. We are often biased in favour of people or groups we see as familiar, making us think of them as being 'safe', and biased against groups we have learned to see as distinct or 'unsafe'. These associations, whether conscious or unconscious, can shape our attitudes and comfort levels around people we perceive as different and can, in turn, affect how we treat them (Box 2.2).

Examples of implicit bias include:

- preferring to socialise with people who only look like you or have similar identities to yours, without noticing that you tend to do this
- reflexively feeling discomfort when you are around individuals or groups with certain characteristics (based on, for example, race, sexual orientation or gender), even though you do not know anything about them as people
- automatically changing how you speak with or about other people who identify differently from you
- regularly showing more respect or giving preferential treatment to certain people based solely on particular characteristics
- having a negative opinion about someone, e.g. assuming someone is unhealthy or unintelligent, based on their race, age, gender or other characteristics, without any personal knowledge of them as an individual.

Box 2.2 **Implicit bias.**

Abdullah Mufti is a postdoctorate Fellow who, having completed his PhD in cancer research, is hoping to further his career by seeking a lectureship position whilst continuing his research. Having had multiple research articles accepted for high-impact journals, he has struggled to find an academic research post. Having written to various institutes, he has either not heard back from them or they have declined to consider his experience within their laboratories. Out of frustration at his lack of progress and curiosity regarding his lack of responses, he changed his name to Duncan Smith. He had prompt replies and was offered several opportunities to pursue with the same institutions that had previously rejected his applications.

Evidence shows that implicit attitudes are widespread amongst populations globally, influencing everyday behaviours. For instance, one widely cited study by Rooth [1] found that simply changing names from White-sounding ones to Black-sounding ones on CVs had a negative effect on shortlisting for interviews. Implicit bias was suspected to be the culprit, and replication of the study in Sweden, using Arab-sounding names instead of Swedish-sounding names, found a correlation between the HR professionals who preferred the CVs with Swedish-sounding names and a higher level of implicit bias towards Arabs.

Explicit bias

Explicit bias is the conscious process by which we evaluate another person or persons, deem them 'acceptable' or 'unacceptable', and then treat them according to how we see them. Unlike implicit bias, which is often unconscious or automatic, explicit bias is making a clear and conscious judgement about groups of people based on their identity.

Examples of explicit bias include:

- consciously using language that is derogatory, disrespectful, a slur or othering when speaking about people with different identities
- reacting angrily or disrespectfully to someone speaking another language (or speaking with a specific accent) or wearing clothing that is significant to their culture, religion or ethnicity because of negative personal feelings about what it means to be part of that culture, religion or ethnicity (Box 2.3)
- treating a person or group of people as unintelligent or immature, or being overtly condescending because of the characteristics of those people (based on, for example, race, sexual orientation or gender)
- bullying or discriminating against people because they are different, either because of your own biases or because you want to belong to the 'in group'.

Box 2.3 **Explicit bias.**

A female Muslim medical student, Salma Shafiq, is on a paediatric placement. She wears the hijab. During this placement, the students receive group teaching about Paediatric Life Support (PLS) from a paediatric consultant.

This teaching session covers the ABCDE assessment of unwell children. The Resuscitation Council UK algorithm advises an assessment of breathing by doing the following:
- **Look** for chest movements.
- **Listen** at the child's nose and mouth for breath sounds.
- **Feel** for air movement on your cheek.

All the students were given an opportunity to practise the algorithm whilst being observed by their peers and the consultant.

After a few students, it is Salma's turn to be observed. Whilst Salma is undertaking the assessment, the consultant stops her and asks how she feels for the breath. She states that she is feeling it on her cheek. The consultant then shouts at her, 'You are supposed to be feeling for it on your ears whilst you listen to the breathing, and you cannot do that with that thing wrapped around your head!' (in reference to her hijab). Feeling embarrassed, Salma responds that she thought she could feel the breath on her cheek, to which the consultant states, 'I will let you off today, but in real life, you need to take that thing off your head and do it properly'. Due to her acute distress and attempt to maintain composure, Salma keeps forgetting how to run the algorithm. The consultant throws a marker pen at her and tells her that she cannot move away from the station until she has completed the algorithm correctly. She eventually manages to do this before leaving the room in tears.

Whilst the Equality Act covers many forms of explicit bias, implicit bias is often a common cause of discrimination, including discriminatory practices in educational institutions, the criminal justice system and workplace practices.

Internalised bias

Sometimes, the harmful messages we hear become part of how we act towards ourselves and people like us – this is internalised bias. For example, a person from a Black or minority ethnic background may have internalised racism. They begin to believe and accept the stereotypes and beliefs about themselves based on their own identity and hold harmful attitudes about others with the same identity (Box 2.4).

Box 2.4 **Internalised bias.**

Zawadi Ashanti is a junior doctor in the acute surgical assessment unit. She has to complete a clerking for a 54-year-old male patient, Oji Olwethu, who has attended with abdominal pain and nausea. This patient has been referred in by his GP due to several attendances with abdominal pain. Mr Olewethu reports that he has had the pain for the last few weeks, and the GP has told him that 'all your blood tests are normal, there is nothing wrong'.

He tells Zawadi that he initially had intermittent dull achy-type pain but now has episodes of severe epigastric pain radiating into his back. He has tried paracetamol and ibuprofen, but this has not been helping. He has not used any paracetamol recently. Zawadi undertakes an examination which is normal. She states that she will discuss this with a senior colleague and come back to him with a plan. A few minutes later, whilst she is with a different patient, the nurse calls her and tells her that 'I can't pronounce that patient's name, but you literally just saw him, and now he is rolling around the bed saying he is in pain – I don't understand how he can be in so much pain so quickly. Can you write him up for some paracetamol?'. Zawadi prescribes paracetamol and returns to her patient. On senior review, Mr Olwethu is referred for a CT scan which reveals pancreatic cancer.

Studies [2,3] outline racial bias in pain assessment and management. Whilst the studies have established bias from White healthcare professionals towards Black, Asian and ethnic minority patients, internalised bias can occur because of systemic racial prejudices.

Internalised bias has powerful negative impacts on a person's mental and physical health. Research shows that people who have internalised racism have an increased risk of anxiety and depression and suffer lower self-esteem levels.

Part of the way our brains make sense of the world is by putting things into categories. The tendency to sort into groups and order these groups is inherent. By age five, children can sort people into groups based on age, gender and race. Of course, this is not enough, in and of itself, to lead to bias.

Racism as an example of bias

Racism can take different forms, including structural, institutional, interpersonal and internalised. It is a system of structuring opportunity and assigning value based on physical properties such as skin colour. This 'system' unfairly disadvantages some individuals and groups and affects an individual's physical health and mental health.

The effects of racism are wide-ranging and include daily interpersonal interactions such as poorer access and poorer outcomes related to healthcare, education and employment. Racism can be seen as an emerging determinant of health and integral to the 'causes of the

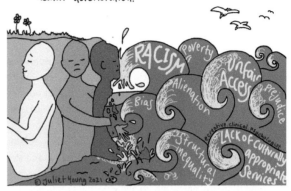

Figure 2.1 Weathering hypothesis for early health deterioration as a result of racism and discrimination.
Source: © Dr Juliet Young, clinical psychologist, permission granted for use within this book.

causes' of the inequalities we see across society. It unfairly advantages individuals belonging to socially and politically dominant racial groups (see Chapter 4).

The 'weathering effect' also explains the premature decline in health outcomes of Black and minority ethnic people exposed to repeated and constant lifelong stressors. Constant exposure to these stressors, underpinned by racism and bias, causes individuals subject to economic and social disadvantages to age prematurely, in both body and mind (Figure 2.1).

Impact of bias in healthcare

Bias can have a significant impact on the way in which clinicians conduct consultations and make decisions for patients. Explicit bias is, by definition, an awareness that an evaluation is taking place. It is often negative implicit bias that is of particular concern within healthcare. Bias built into policies and processes can place patients at risk and, in some cases, can harm patients. The lack of awareness of implicit bias can perpetuate systemic inequalities and lead to inaccurate diagnoses for people with darker skin tones (Box 2.5).

Box 2.5 **Impact of bias in healthcare.**

Kofi Omari is a young professional of African descent. Lately, Kofi has been feeling fatigued and getting more headaches than usual. He notices a rash on his lower back where the skin, normally an even brown, is darker and slightly purple-tinged in some areas.

The first doctor Kofi consults sends him home with a prescription for a steroid cream, which seems to do nothing. Weeks later, the discolouration finally fades, but Kofi's muscles ache and he feels depleted, such that he has to take sick leave from work. Kofi consults another doctor who guesses that he has chronic fatigue syndrome.

Kofi feels sick for months before consulting yet another physician, who finally runs the right tests and correctly informs Kofi that he has Lyme disease.

Early diagnosis and treatment are critical for Lyme disease. But the first physician Kofi saw did not consider that Kofi's rash might be due to Lyme disease because they had been trained to look for a red-and-pink skin colouration for this disease. That is not what Lyme typically looks like on Black skin.

Since the Black Lives Matter movement, many institutions may consider implementing bias training to help mitigate racism. However, awareness of implicit bias or tokenistic bias training must not deflect from the broader socioeconomic, political and structural barriers that individuals face.

Similarly, implicit bias should not be used to avoid responsibility or ignore explicit bias that may favour perpetuating prejudice and stereotypes. Training in this field should not reflect a tick-box online exercise but should be designed practically to allow people to interact, debate, understand and evolve in their individual and collective thinking.

A 2019 study by Obermeyer et al. [4] (Box 2.6) noted racism in decision-making software used by US hospitals. The researchers concluded that the algorithm was less likely to refer Black people than White people who were equally sick to programmes that aim to improve care for patients with complex medical needs.

Box 2.6 **Health system biases.**

Health systems rely on commercial prediction algorithms to identify and help patients with complex health needs. Obermeyer et al. [4] showed that a widely used algorithm affecting millions of patients exhibits significant racial bias. At a given risk score, Black patients are considerably sicker than White patients, as evidenced by signs of uncontrolled illnesses. Remedying this disparity would increase the percentage of Black patients receiving additional help from 17.7% to 46.5%. The bias arises because the algorithm predicts healthcare costs rather than illness, but unequal access to care means less money is spent caring for Black patients than White patients. Therefore, despite healthcare cost appearing to be an effective proxy for health by some measures of predictive accuracy, significant racial biases still exist.

Bias in healthcare is not just concerned with those at the receiving end of healthcare; it also affects those that deliver care. It can manifest in several ways, including differential attainment, lower pay for clinicians from ethnic minorities, and a lack of Black surgeons in senior positions (Box 2.7).

Box 2.7 **Race equality in the medical workforce in England – summary findings [5].**

Compared to the overall proportion of doctors in the NHS, Black, Asian and ethnic minority doctors are underrepresented in consultant grade roles but overrepresented in other doctor grades and doctors in postgraduate training. Black, Asian and ethnic minority doctors are also underrepresented in academic positions.

Black, Asian and ethnic minority doctors report a worse experience than their White colleagues regarding harassment, bullying, abuse and discrimination from other staff.

Black, Asian and ethnic minority doctors have a worse experience regarding examinations (medical school and postgraduation examinations) and regulation (revalidation, referrals/complaints to GMC, Annual Review of Competence Progression). This discrimination begins early in the career, with Black, Asian and ethnic minority students less likely to attain a place in medical school than White students.

Understanding personal bias can help identify judgements made during recruitment processes and help build representative leadership and workforce in the healthcare system of the population they serve. This is likely to help deliver better patient care, outcomes and safety.

Other strategies to decrease the impact of bias include using objective criteria to recruit, blind evaluations and salary disclosures. Additional measures include providing an audited system of reporting discrimination, measuring outcomes such as employee recruitment, pay and progression opportunities, and routinely measuring employee perceptions of inclusion and fairness. Such measures are fundamental to help mitigate inequality and associated adversity.

Impact of bias in medical research and policy

To understand ethnic health inequalities and establish policies to improve the health of all people and communities, research must include suitable sampling designs and ensure representative samples of ethnic minority people. While medical research and policy continue to march ahead, it is often unchecked for potential bias. There is a justified argument that these issues have compounded inequalities further [6].

Bias in medical research can undermine efficient scientific discovery and efforts to improve patient outcomes. We see, time and time again, medical research that excludes diverse community participation. It is, therefore, no surprise that interventions and policies developed as a result of such biased research do not meet the needs of all populations (Box 2.8). For example, the underdetection of hypoxaemia by pulse oximetry [7,8] and the underdiagnosis of melanomas by cancer software in Black patients result from White patients being used as the default group in the algorithms used to develop and test these medical devices. This was also exemplified by the COVID-19 pandemic, highlighting the ever-growing concerns and evidence base for the ethnic disparity in medical research among ethnic minority communities [6].

Box 2.8 **Racial bias in pulse oximetry.**

During the COVID-19 pandemic, Sjoding and colleagues [7] compared almost 11 000 pairs of oxygen saturation measurements with pulse oximetry and arterial blood gas among Black and White patients. Black patients were 8–11% (relative risk three times) more likely to have lower arterial saturation when compared with pulse oximetry for White patients. This has clear implications for people's care and self-care during health challenges such as COVID-19 and general respiratory conditions.

A rapid review of racial bias in pulse oximetry, carried out by the NHS Race and Health Observatory in England, led to the UK government commissioning an independent review of bias across medical devices and assessments, as well as further research in this area [8].

Rather than counteracting discriminatory processes of wider society, healthcare systems can often mirror the influences that undermine the health of ethnic minority people and underserved populations, for example, as a result of bias in testing and diagnoses [9]. Bias in research and policy contributes to this unwanted situation. Getting this right will not just benefit ethnic minority people – debiasing medical research and policy will benefit everyone.

Tackling bias

The first step toward countering any form of bias is acknowledging its existence. Tackling interpersonal bias, therefore, has a critical role to play.

Tackling or unlearning biases can be a prolonged process, not least because biases can often be deeply embedded within our society and because discrimination happens every day in big and small ways (macro- and microaggressions). A macroaggression is a racist act directed at everyone of the same race, gender or group. Individuals spreading misinformation about COVID-19 and blaming Asia are examples of macroaggression. As a result, there has been an increase in hate crimes against Asians [10]. Microaggressions are defined as everyday, subtle, intentional – and frequently unintentional – interactions or behaviours that communicate a bias toward historically marginalised groups. The distinction between microaggressions and overt discrimination or macroaggressions is that people who commit microaggressions may be unaware of their actions. It should be acknowledged that aggressions, whether 'macro' or 'micro', have debilitating impacts on the recipient.

It is not easy to unlearn biases, but it is important to do so for our mental health, relationships with others and the betterment of society. Some common, helpful actions can be taken to identify and unlearn biases.

- *Check implicit biases*: one way to check your own biases is to imagine people in different occupations. What do you see when you imagine a nurse, a teacher or a lawyer? Seeing where your brain goes automatically can help you unpack what you assume about others based on little information.
- *Demonstrate empathy*: once you are aware of your biases, learning how they can impact others is an integral part of practising empathy. Such concern for others can help motivate you to learn more about more extensive systems of discrimination.
- *Replace biases*: actively imagining someone you have stereotyped as the opposite of that stereotype can help to reorient a person to have fewer implicit biases. Actively deciding to replace stereotypical thinking can help rebuild thoughts in the long term.
- *Educate and inform*: discrimination often stems from ignorance. Learning about or experiencing other cultures, ethnicities and identities can help unlearn biases and appreciate the strength of people's differences.

Conclusion

Bias is part of how human beings process information. Bias can often lead to discriminatory practices, which, in the area of health and care, can place certain people, such as ethnic minorities, at risk. Such biases should be challenged at their root cause. However, to do so, we need to be honest, acknowledge the existence of that bias and work towards tackling it head on. Interventions that focus on the causes of the bias are fundamental to help mitigate inequality and associated adversity.

Further reading/resources

Adebowale, V. and Rao, M. (2020) Racism in medicine: why equality matters to all. *BMJ*, **368**, m530.

Atewologun, D., Cornish, T. and Tresh, F. (2018) Unconscious bias: training. Equality and Human Rights Commission. www.equalityhumanrights.com/en/publication-download/unconscious-bias-training-assessment-evidence-effectiveness (accessed September 2022)

Bertrand, M. and Mullainathan, S. (2004) Are Emily and Greg more employable than Lakisha and Jamal? A field experiment on labour market discrimination. *American Economic Review*, **94**, 991–1013.

Blair, I.V., Steiner, J.F. and Havranek, E.P. (2011) Unconscious (implicit) bias and health disparities: where do we go from here? *Permanente Journal*, **15**, 71–78.

Gale, M., Pieterse, A., Lee, D., Huynh, K., Powell, S. and Kirkinis, K. (2020) A meta-analysis of the relationship between internalized racial oppression and health-related outcomes. *Counseling Psychology*, **48**, 498–525.

References

1 Rooth, D.O. (2010) Automatic associations and discrimination in hiring: real world evidence. *Labour Economics*, **17** (3), 523–534.

2 Hoffman, K.M., Trawalter, S., Axt, J.R. and Oliver, M.N. (2016) Racial bias in pain assessment and treatment recommendations, and false beliefs about biological differences between blacks and whites. *Proceedings of the National Academy of Sciences USA*, **113** (16), 4296–4301.

3 Trawalter, S. and Hoffman, K.M. (2015) Got pain? Racial bias in perceptions of pain. *Social and Personality Psychologgy Compass*, **9** (3), 146–157.

4 Obermeyer, Z., Powers, B., Vogeli, C. and Mullainathan, S. (2019) Dissecting racial bias in an algorithm used to manage the health of populations. *Science*, **366** (6464), 447–453.

5 NHS England (2021) Medical Workforce Race Equality Standard (MWRES): WRES indicators for the medical workforce 2020. www.england.nhs.uk/wp-content/uploads/2021/07/MWRES-DIGITAL-2020_FINAL.pdf

6 Powell, R.A., Njoku, C., Elangovan, R. et al. (2022) Tackling racism in UK health research. *BMJ*, **376**, e065574.

7 Sjoding, M.W., Dickson, R.P., Iwashyna, T.J. et al. (2020) Racial bias in pulse oximetry measurement. *New England Journal of Medicine*, **383** (25), 2477–2478.

8 NHS Race and Health Observatory (2021) Pulse oximetry and racial bias: recommendations for national healthcare, regulatory and research bodies www.nhsrho.org/wp-content/uploads/2021/03/Pulse-oximetry-racial-bias-report.pdf.

9 Gopal, D.P., Chetty, U., O'Donnell, P. et al. (2021) Implicit bias in healthcare: clinical practice, research and decision making. *Future Healthcare Journal*, **8** (1), 40–48.

10 Gray, C. and Hansen, K. (2021) Did Covid-19 lead to an increase in hate crimes toward Chinese people in London? *Journal of Contemporary Criminal Justice*, **37** (4), 569–588.

CHAPTER 3

Racism in Healthcare

Olivia King[1] and Anton Emmanuel[2]

[1] Senior Strategy and Policy Lead, NHS England, England
[2] Professor and Consultant Neurogastroenterologist, UCL, UCLH and NHNN, Lead of the Workforce Race Equality Standard, NHS England, Interim Joint Director of Equality, Diversity and Inclusion, NHS England, University College London Hospitals, England

---

OVERVIEW

- Discrimination, racism and cultural insensitivity persist in healthcare organisations in the UK.
- Minority ethnic patients report fewer good experiences than White British patients in almost every dimension of general practice services.
- Minority ethnic people are overrepresented in the NHS workforce proportionate to population figures but experience persistent inequalities in experience and career development compared to their White peers.
- Only 10% of NHS Trust board members in England are from minority ethnic groups, and more than two-fifths of NHS Trusts have no minority ethnic board members.
- Over the past decade, national race health reports in the UK have been united in recommending improvement in data collection and analysis to support evidence-based interventions to address race inequalities for patients and staff.

Introduction

The National Health Service (NHS) was established in 1948 and is the world's most widely recognised healthcare institution. It was a core component of the major social reforms after the Second World War. Race discrimination permeates all aspects of healthcare culture, operations and structure. There are similar experiences in Continental European countries, the USA, Canada and Australia. Racism is a recognised social determinant of health and perpetuates ethnic inequities in healthcare outcomes, access and delivery [1]. This has negative consequences for patients, carers and healthcare workers, leading to a higher risk of illness and, in some cases, lower standards of care for people based on their race or perceived race (see Box 3.1).

Box 3.1 **Definitions.**

Race is a historical, social construct of difference which informs social practices, shapes institutions and affects the distribution of resources. Defining racial groups is challenging and often informed by conflict. Different legislative frameworks can be used to challenge racial discrimination. The most significant is the Equality Act 2010, which states that you must not be discriminated against because of your race, where race can mean colour, nationality, citizenship, ethnicity and national origins.

Individual racism involves holding race-based values to inform choices and behaviours (e.g. refusing to be treated by a Muslim doctor and using derogatory language).

Institutional racism is the collective failure of an organisation to provide an appropriate and professional service to people because of their colour, culture or ethnic origin. It can be seen or detected in processes, attitudes and behaviour, which amount to discrimination through unwitting prejudice, ignorance, thoughtlessness and racial stereotyping.

Systemic/structural racism is the alienation of specific groups from positions of authority, power and access to resources by customs, cultures and ideology. In the workplace, this manifests as modes of discrimination that can determine who gets hired, trained, promoted, retained, demoted and fired. This form of racism contributes to maintaining a sociocultural and political economic system that creates and reproduces race inequality.

Microaggressions are subtle, indirect and sometimes everyday exchanges that undermine and denigrate a marginalised group. This can include a statement or action which marginalises and dehumanises a person in a way that is hard to describe, use as evidence and pin down. In the workplace, this might manifest as a 'joke' about someone's race, using derogatory signifiers aligned with stereotypes or denying the existence of racism.

Racial trauma results from racism, racist bias, exposure to racist microaggressions and observing others being subjected to racism. It can affect all aspects of a person's life and cause similar symptoms to post-traumatic stress disorder. It can lead to people avoiding accessing services, including healthcare, when needed. It often results in healthcare staff leaving the service. Racial trauma has been recognised globally to affect a person's socioeconomic outcomes and health status profoundly. When others deny that trauma exists or blame the victim, it may intensify the trauma.

Emotional labour is used to talk about how workers manage their feelings and emotions about the organisational rules, guidelines and experiences. Emotional labour results in individuals having to suppress feelings to sustain an outward appearance that fits their job's requirements. Regarding race, research has shown that emotional labour is a burden borne by minority ethnic staff due to their fears

---

ABC of Equality, Diversity and Inclusion in Healthcare, First Edition. Edited by Shehla Imtiaz-Umer and John Frain.
© 2023 John Wiley & Sons Ltd. Published 2023 by John Wiley & Sons Ltd.

of adverse consequences for their employment should they be seen engaged in discussing racism, reporting it or challenging it. Emotional labour is also experienced when caring for overtly or indirectly racist patients, as healthcare staff are bound by a duty of providing equal care for all patients as expressed in healthcare institutional regulations. Strategies to manage emotional labour described by staff include working harder to prove their competence and faking, blocking or hiding their emotions when they encounter racism. Research has shown that medical students have similar experiences and that both staff and students lack suitable psychologically safe spaces to discuss, share and develop techniques to manage this.

Sources: Equality and Human Rights Commission (UK) on defining terminology from the Equality Act 2010.

Ahlberg, B.M., Hamed, S., Bradby, H., Moberg, C. and Thapar-Björkert, S. (2022) 'Just throw it behind you and just keep going': emotional labor when ethnic minority healthcare staff encounter racism in healthcare. *Frontiers in Sociology*. www.frontiersin.org/articles/10.3389/fsoc.2021.741202

Cabinet Office Race Disparity Unit. www.gov.uk/government/organisations/race-disparity-unit.

Although race in healthcare research is primarily US based, the UK government has recognised the need for comprehensive data management and interrogation systems and analysis for understanding and tackling health disparities based on race. This is similarly the case in Continental Europe, with research largely led by the European Commission, which recommends improvements in data and analysis in all member states to ensure race discrimination is identified, monitored and tackled [2]. In the UK, most research has been on maternal and infant care, cardiovascular disease, diabetes and access to GP services. All these areas show a consistent disparity in experience and outcome by race [3,4]. Data about ethnic health disparities are derived from health records in the UK. A specific area of concern has been maternal and infant mortality (Box 3.2).

Box 3.2 **Examples of race disparities in maternal and infant mortality.**

Infant and maternal mortality rates are higher among Black African and South Asian groups. Compared with the White population, the rate of women dying in the UK in 2016–2018 during or up to one year after pregnancy is more than four times higher in the Black population and almost double in the Asian population. In response, the Department of Health and Social Care published 'Safer maternity care: progress and next steps' with recommendations for improved data collection, training and development for the workforce and rigorous investigations for improvement. NHS England launched the National Maternity Transformation Programme to reduce disparities and infant and maternal mortality rates by 2025.

Sources: White, C. (2021) Ethnic differences in life expectancy and mortality from selected causes in England and Wales: 2011 to 2014. www.ons.gov.uk/peoplepopulationandcommunity/birthsdeath sandmarriages/lifeexpectancies/articles/ethnicdifferencesinlifeexpec tancyandmortalityfromselectedcausesinenglandandwales/2011to2014

Department of Health and Social Care (2017) Safer maternity care: progress and next steps. https://assets.publishing.service.gov.uk/government/uploads/system/uploads/attachment_data/file/662969/Safer_maternity_care_-_progress_and_next_steps.pdf.

However, the quality of information is not standardised and is incomplete. Data on mortality by ethnic group are unavailable because ethnicity is not recorded on death registration in England and Wales (it was introduced in Scotland in 2012). Currently, analyses of mortality are based on the country of birth of migrants as a reference for ethnicity, but this excludes second-generation migrants. Public health teams in England have begun to link death records with secondary sources to derive ethnicity and outcome information. However, the data remain limited and pose barriers to understanding and addressing health disparities by race.

Race discrimination has taken on a higher profile since 2019. It has increasingly become the focus of national strategies due to the cost to population health and overhauling a dated healthcare model. The COVID-19 pandemic drew attention to this with a higher death rate and risk of dying of people from minority groups than the majority White population (Box 3.3). Due to the pandemic, the UK government has stated it will introduce ethnicity recording on death certificates.

Box 3.3 **Race disparities: COVID-19 pandemic.**

Between 8 December 2020 and 12 June 2021, people from all ethnic minority groups (except the Chinese group and women in the White other ethnic groups) had higher rates of death involving COVID-19 than the White British population.

The rate of death involving COVID-19 was highest for the Bangladeshi ethnic group (5.0 times greater than the White British group for males and 4.5 times greater for females), followed by the Pakistani (3.1 for males, 2.6 for females) and Black African (2.4 for males, 1.7 for females) ethnic groups.

Government figures show that since the COVID-19 vaccination programme began, the risk of death from COVID-19 has remained higher in minority ethnic groups than in the White British ethnic group.

Analysis by Public Health England of survival among confirmed cases revealed that after accounting for sex, age, deprivation and region, people of Bangladeshi ethnicity had twice the risk of death compared to White British people, and those of Chinese, Indian, Pakistani, other Asian, Caribbean and other Black ethnicity had between 10% and 50% higher risk of death when compared to White British people.

Sources: BMA (2022) COVID-19: analysing the impact of coronavirus on doctors. www.bma.org.uk/advice-and-support/covid-19/what-the-bma-is-doing/covid-19-analysing-the-impact-of-coronavirus-on-doctors

Office for National Statistics (2022) Updating ethnic contrasts in deaths involving the coronavirus (COVID-19), England: 8 December 2020 to 1 December 2021. www.ons.gov.uk/peoplepopulationand community/birthsdeathsandmarriages/deaths/articles/updatingethniccontrastsindeathsinvolvingthecoronavirus covid19englandandwales/8december2020to1december2021

Kursumovic, E., Lennane, S. and Cook, T.M. (2020) Deaths in healthcare workers due to COVID-19: the need for robust data and analysis. *Anaesthesia*, **75**(8), 989–992.

Public Health England (2020) *Disparities in the Risk and Outcomes of COVID-19*. London: PHE.

Racism in healthcare is highly complex. There are multiple and convergent issues: discrimination and harassment of staff based on race; disempowering minority population groups and communities in their ability to maintain optimum health through life; inequitable service delivery to people because of their race and/or perceived race; bias in medical research and education (Box 3.4).

Box 3.4 **Racism in healthcare: general practice.**

National surveys show that experience of care varies across ethnicities and within ethnic groups (by variables including income, residency, disability and gender) and, in general, contributes to poorer and differential outcomes across different care pathways compared with the White population. The issue is complex and intersects with poverty, deprivation and access to GP services. Minority ethnic groups are more likely to live in deprived areas, which are less likely to have a suitable number of GP services and are more likely to be serviced by minority ethnic-led GP which have fewer personnel and resources. Furthermore, general practices led by minority ethnic GPs report that CQC inspectors are less likely to understand the healthcare challenges that minority ethnic patients and staff face.

Three mechanisms are considered to produce and reproduce discriminatory patterns of healthcare. The first is bias (including prejudice) against minority population groups, the second is historically driven clinical uncertainty when interacting with minority patient groups, and the third is the beliefs (including negative social stereotypes) held about the health of minority groups. Patients have also been found to react to providers' behaviour, contributing to aversion to using services when needed, thereby putting people at higher risk of developing long-term conditions.

Sources: The King's Fund (2021) *The Health of People from Ethnic Minority Groups in England*. London: King's Fund.

Marmot, M. (2020) Health Equity in England: The Marmot Review 10 Years On. www.health.org.uk/publications/reports/the-marmot-review-10-years-on

Care Quality Commission (2021) *Ethnic Minority-Led GP Practices: Impact and Experience of CQC Regulation*. London: CQC.

Casual clinical stereotypes cause bias in decision making, leading to missed diagnoses, delayed treatment and preventable outcomes. This is compounded by other forms of discrimination, including disability, gender, religion or belief and sexual orientation (Box 3.5). Eliminating racism in healthcare must tackle broader issues of discrimination and exclusion for multiple groups that have been represented poorly in medical education, healthcare research and policies, processes and strategies.

Box 3.5 **Examples of racism in healthcare.**

'They feel that (nurses) do not want to bother them. They are not wanted. They feel that nurses do not like them. Sometimes, what nurses do is not obvious, but it is underhand. Those (patients) who cannot speak English get into trouble, and they get a bit bullied as well.' Pakistani patient in the UK

'To be honest, some patients have a chip on their shoulder about colour, and a lot of fuss is made up over nothing … I am sorry to say.' White registered nurse caring for Pakistani patients in the UK

'I have interpreted for Somali patients because I speak Somali. And many times, as an interpreter, I am not allowed to say anything, or I am not allowed to have an opinion … I stopped interpreting because I see how these people are treated in healthcare.' Midwife of Somali heritage supporting White colleagues to deliver care in Sweden.

Sources: Cortis J.D. (2004) Meeting the needs of minority ethnic patients. *Journal of Advanced Nursing*, **48**(1), 51–58.

Cortis, J.D. (2000) Perceptions and experiences with nursing care: a study of Pakistani (Urdu) communities in the United Kingdom. *Journal of Transcultural Nursing*, **11**(2), 111–118.

Historical context

The NHS is the largest employer in Europe and relies on a workforce drawn from all over the world. Excluding the primary care and community workforce, 85.4% of NHS staff in England are British, with 5.8% reporting nationality from an Asian country and 5.4% from a European Union nationality. The proportion of internationally trained healthcare workers varies across regions. In London, 27% of staff report a non-British nationality. In the North East and Yorkshire, the proportion is 7% (Table 3.1)

The number of staff from Africa, Asia and South-East Asia has risen since 2016. This trend is expected to continue with the shortfall in local staff, lack of uptake of training spaces and problems with retaining current staff (Figure 3.1).

Current disparities in healthcare are rooted in history. British and European colonial ideology specifically used pseudo-science (Box 3.6) and medical experimentation to empirically justify the subjugation of people across the globe and deepen colonial incursion into sovereign territories [5,6].

Box 3.6 **Examples of pseudo-science.**

An example of pseudo-science was when ethnologists with little formal training reported on different groups of people, and these observations were used to classify different races into hierarchies. This process was considered scientific even though skin colour was often the element used to rank races, with lighter-skinned humans considered superior. In the process, there was no evaluation by European scientists of the capabilities of Europeans themselves. Therefore, the scientific observations were based on the predetermined notion of European superiority, as demonstrated in the work of influential scientists across Western economies of the time, such as Francis Galton (1892) and Charles Darwin (1871).

Table 3.1 NHS Trusts nationalities.

Most common nationalities of NHS staff			
UK/British	1,118,116	Spanish	5,405
Indian	32,117	Romanian	5,251
Filipino	25,423	Pakistani	4,902
Irish	14,151	Zimbabwean	4,780
Polish	10,520	Ghanaian	3,395
Nigerian	10,494	Greek	3,348
Portuguese	7,831	Egyptian	2,895
Italian	6,660	Malaysian	2,581

Source: House of Commons Library, NHS Staff from Overseas Statistics, 2021.

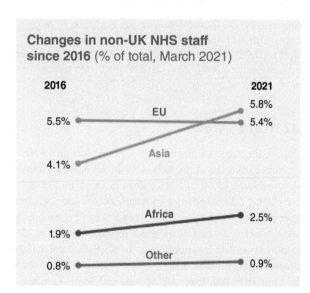

Changes in non-UK NHS staff since 2016 (% of total, March 2021)

	2016	2021
EU	5.5%	5.8%
Asia	4.1%	5.4%
Africa	1.9%	2.5%
Other	0.8%	0.9%

Figure 3.1 Chart illustrating changes in non-UK NHS staff since 2016 (% of total).
Source: House of Commons Library, NHS Staff from Overseas Statistics, 2021.

Other examples include the production of racial biology in the nineteenth century by Swedish scientists, including Carl Linnaeus of Sweden, who divided humans into four distinct races, and Anders Retzius, who developed methods of measuring the skull of different races.

In the USA, epidemiological studies were used to justify slavery as a state in which Black people were free of worry and mental illness, which was beneficial because if they were set free, they would become mentally ill.

Source: Ahlberg, B.M., Hamed, S., Bradby, H., Moberg, C. and Thapar-Björkert, S. (2022) 'Just throw it behind you and just keep going': emotional labor when ethnic minority healthcare staff encounter racism in healthcare. *Frontiers in Sociology*. www.frontiersin.org/articles/10.3389/fsoc.2021.741202

and authors, with the rest of the world continuing to be dependent on it for scientific direction, validation and aid. This is argued by scholars of medical history [7]. They seek to challenge and interrogate the foundations of race-driven scientific decision making with flawed underpinnings, albeit less overt than during the colonial era.

Hierarchical rendering of 'race groups' was used to justify and perpetuate experiments on people of colour. This continues to affect trust between the medical profession and minority ethnic groups in Western economies [8] (Box 3.7).

Box 3.7 **Race-based experiments.**

Notable examples of race-based experiments include those by J. Marion Sims in the mid-nineteenth century. He experimented on enslaved Black women using unethical practices in the name of gynaecology. None of the women were given pain medication or anaesthesia for invasive procedures.

The Tuskegee study run between 1932 and 1970 deliberately infected Black men in the US with syphilis, leaving them with the disease even after effective treatment became available.

The Rawalpindi experiments (1930s and 1940s) involved the use of mustard gas carried out by British scientists and doctors from Porton Down on hundreds of soldiers from the British Indian Army. These experiments were carried out before and during the Second World War in a military installation at Rawalpindi in modern-day Pakistan.

These examples are just some of those that have come to light. During decolonisation, records and documents were destroyed (termed 'Operation Legacy'), which means we do not have a complete picture of the scale and extent of these experiments in the former colonies and even in the USA.

Sources: Schiebinger, L. *Secret Cures of Slaves: People, Plants, and Medicine in the Eighteenth-Century Atlantic World*. Stanford, CA: Stanford University Press, 2017.
Sato, S. (2017) 'Operation Legacy': Britain's destruction and concealment of colonial records worldwide. *Journal of Imperial and Commonwealth History*, **45**(4), 697–719.

These are examples of how pseudo-science was deployed across history to justify Western interests' sociopolitical and economic hegemony. This crucial underpinning of the ascendancy of Western European perspectives continues to inform medical and broader scientific research, evidenced by the domination of Western academic journals

The legacy of the experiments and theories from this period continues to underpin racist assumptions and racialised healthcare policies, facilitated by the paucity of coverage of race and history in most educational establishments. They have led to current racialised healthcare practices. The most notable and well researched include the assumption that Black women do not need pain medication in similar situations to White women [9] (Box 3.8).

Box 3.8 How painful is it?

A 47-year-old man of West African origin presented to the emergency department with acute abdominal pain. He had no relevant past history and worked as a bus driver. He was in severe pain but not given any pain relief beyond paracetamol because a member of A&E staff mistook him for another Black patient who was a 'morphine seeker'. His ultrasound excluded gallstones and he was discharged home on more paracetamol. His blood tests showed slight anaemia, but this was presumed to be because he had sickle cell trait (although the patient gave no such history).

Over the next eight days he re-presented three times and on each occasion was discharged home with low-grade analgesia. By now, he was also complaining of pain in his shoulder and spine; no X-rays were taken as his notes now documented that he was an analgesic abuser. He had not been able to work over this period but took himself to the bus depot on day 10 and while driving experienced such severe pain that he had to pull over and was taken by ambulance to a different hospital. He underwent an abdominal CT scan and an X-ray of his shoulder. A diagnosis of primary liver cancer (two lesions 2.2 cm in size) with metastases to the shoulder and spine was made (ultrasound misses up to 20% of such lesions).

Black people are often considered impervious to pain because of their race. Black patients are 22% less likely than White ones to receive appropriate pain relief. This relates to systematised false beliefs amongst up to 50% of White medical staff about the supposed greater pain tolerance of Black people. In addition, those White doctors who reported these beliefs rated Black patients' pain as of lower severity than White patients and made racially biased prescription recommendations.

Source: Trawalter, S. and Hoffman, K.M. (2015) Got pain? Racial bias in perceptions of pain. *Social and Personality Psychology Compass*, **9**(3), 146–157.

Racialised approaches and theories have led to the 'invisibility' of diverse participants in medical technology development and research. For example, the spirometer, a standard medical device used worldwide, measures lung capacity. Still, when first used, doctors felt that Black people had inferior bodies and that White people had higher lung capacity. Even today, spirometers are usually 'race corrected' [10].

Racialised healthcare

Historical framing of White superiority has produced racialised healthcare structures and practices which routinely place White people at an advantage while producing adverse outcomes for people of colour (Box 3.9). The disadvantage is not uniform across the racialised minorities, although it pervades all aspects of healthcare, including research, commissioning, implementation, public consultation, action planning and long-term strategic policy.

Box 3.9 Racialised healthcare.

- False beliefs and race bias about biological differences between Black people and White people in pain perception and treatment recommendation accuracy mean that Black people are less likely to be believed, more likely to have their pain dismissed and less likely to receive the treatment needed in pain management. Black women are five times more likely to die during childbirth, and Asian women are twice as likely to die during childbirth compared with White women in the UK.
- South Asian women have been dismissed by doctors who claim they are suffering from the so-called 'Mrs Bibi syndrome', also known as 'Begum syndrome', referring to an imagined condition where South Asian women are said to exaggerate their health complaints.
- Clinical education lacks diverse training on what skin manifestation of pathological conditions looks like in skin of different tones. People are not taught what cyanosis looks like in Black patients, and skin pigmentation can affect pulse oximeters.
- Persistent and compulsory admission of Black people to psychiatric wards with greater use of security and force. Black adults were more likely than adults in other ethnic groups to have been sectioned under the Mental Health Act.
- Minority ethnic people diagnosed with cancer see their GP several times more than White British people before they are referred to a hospital.

Sources: Raleigh, V. and Holmes, J. (2021) The health of people from ethnic minority groups in England. www.kingsfund.org.uk/publications/health-people-ethnic-minority-groups-england
Marmot, M. (2020) Health Equity in England: The Marmot Review 10 Years On. www.health.org.uk/publications/reports/the-marmot-review-10-years-on
Fazil, Q. (2018) *Cancer and Black and Minority Ethnic Communities*. London: Race Equality Foundation.

Anti-Blackness: wider implications of racism in healthcare

Anti-Black racism is rooted in the history and experience of enslavement and is targeted against people of African descent and heritage [11]. This has implications for patients and Black healthcare professionals. One reason why Black clinicians remain unable to break through to leadership positions of power and influence is the production and reproduction of anti-Black racism [11] (Box 3.10).

Box 3.10 Anti-Blackness: wider implications of racism in healthcare.

Hoffman et al. reviewed decision making by race. They found that in hospital settings, clinicians who perceived Black people to be biologically different were more likely to rate the pain of Black patients as lower than comparable White patients and provide poorer treatment options for Black patients (Box 3.11). Other studies have found that Black patients report better health outcomes, satisfaction, communication and medical adherence when receiving treatment from a Black clinician, which has led to calls for an increase in the representation of Black clinicians in healthcare.

Anti-Blackness remains pervasive in medical academia and education as it is ubiquitous in all socioeconomic, cultural and policy elements. It underpins how people of African heritage are profiled and treated by public authorities not just in the UK but across other Western democracies, including Australia, Canada, France, New Zealand and the USA. Further information is in the Lammy Review (2017), which examined various countries' evidence.

Sources: Hoffman, K.M., Trawalter, S., Axt, J.R. and Oliver, M.N. (2016) Racial bias in pain assessment and treatment recommendations, and false beliefs about biological differences between blacks and whites. *Proceedings of the National Academy of Sciences*, **113**(16), 4296–4301.

Alsan, M., Garrick, O. and Graziani G. (2019) Does diversity matter for health? Experimental evidence from Oakland. *American Economic Review*, **109**(12), 4071–4111.

Box 3.11 **Sickle cell disease inequity.**

Sickle cell disease is an inherited blood disorder that primarily affects Black people, and the most common clinical manifestation is acute severe crises requiring hospitalisation. Sickle cell patients frequently receive substandard care, with significant variations in care depending on which staff are on duty or which hospital the patient is in. Consequent to the low levels of awareness and training in sickle cell, patients often feel as though they are not treated as a priority by healthcare professionals, which relates to racial prejudice. Sickle cell services are underresourced and understaffed, and there has been a lack of investment in sickle cell research over decades.

Source: All-Party Parliamentary Group (2021) No one's listening: an inquiry into the avoidable deaths and failures of care for sickle cell patients in secondary care. www.sicklecellsociety.org/wp-content/uploads/2021/11/No-Ones-Listening-PDF-Final.pdf.

UK guidance on treating high blood pressure recommends angiotensin-converting enzyme inhibitors for everyone except people of Black African or Black Caribbean heritage, who are advised to start calcium channel blockers.

The underdiagnosis of melanomas by cancer software in Black patients is a direct result of White patients being used as the default group in algorithms used to develop and test medical devices. The setting of research agendas and priorities is far from racially neutral or objective. Across healthcare infrastructure, agendas and priorities are influenced by multiple interlinked biases.

The National Institution of Health Research (NIHR) in the UK reported that research with minority applicants lags far behind. Diversity is not embedded in research decision making [12]. Although these biases' damaging implications in healthcare are gradually being acknowledged, investment in improvement is lacking and threatens future representative healthcare in medical devices and technological development.

Staff experiences

When the NHS was founded, it was in a unique position. The British Empire was prolific and, at its height, commanded more than 22% of the global land mass and 23% of the global population. There was a ready supply of workers to rebuild the country after the Second World War. People from British colonies were recruited to build the institution but denied fundamental equality or recognition of their skills, as evidenced by the Windrush Generation [13]. There were less than two weeks between the docking of the *Empire Windrush* at Tilbury on 22nd June 1948 and the launch of the NHS on 5th July that same year.

The establishment of the NHS coincided with the partition of India in 1947, leading to over 55 000 people who lost homes and jobs coming to Britain, some of whom worked for the NHS [14]. The Willink Committee of 1957 cut spaces for medical students while ignoring the rise in UK population numbers. This led to the targeted recruitment of doctors from Sri Lanka, India, Pakistan and Bangladesh. By the 1950s, the Asian doctor population was estimated to be 3000. UK-trained doctors, unhappy with the reduced pay due to the establishment of a national service, left to work in Canada and the USA – with an estimated 3500 leaving the country. By 1971, 18 000 doctors had been recruited from Pakistan and India. Over 30% of the doctors in the NHS in England were internationally trained in educational institutions that British colonial administrations had established in their countries of birth. This is another reason for the unique position of the NHS and the perpetuation of race-based ideology in medical academia – the doctors were trained to the standards, with similar frames of reference and theoretical underpinnings aligned to the medical and educational imperatives of the UK.

International recruitment was the chosen solution when nursing vacancies spiralled at different points in NHS history. In 1998, for example, 8000 nursing vacancies were filled by overseas nurses [14]. Difficulty retaining the internationally trained workforce is documented by the lack of adjustments for cultural inclusion, language support and wider global concerns about healthcare worker shortages in other parts of the world.

In 1999, a directive by the World Health Organization was issued to monitor global medical and nursing supply and to create lists of banned countries for recruitment [15]. This has now become known as the WHO Global Code of Practice on the International Recruitment of Health Personnel [16]. At the same time, those who came to work in the UK were often relegated to fields that were not their first choice, and the aspirations of these doctors and nurses were not met. Most of those who came to the country to work saw it as an opportunity to upskill and continue their learning journey, but that was not how the NHS perceived them [14].

General practice is an area of healthcare dominated by internationally trained doctors, especially in inner cities and areas of poverty and deprivation. These locations were left without practitioners following the exodus of White doctors at the establishment of the NHS. Even before the NHS, doctors of Black and Asian heritage set up practices in areas that were neglected by others [17].

Workforce Race Equality Standard

Because of inconsistent organisational action to tackle racism in the workplace and to explore the scope and extent of the problem, the Workforce Race Equality Standard (WRES) was mandated in April 2015.

Using a collection of nine indicators (four from the annual NHS Staff Survey, four from employee records and one from board composition), the WRES provides a check of where the NHS is in terms of representation and experience of Black and minority ethnic (BME) staff compared to their White colleagues. The indicators also demonstrate organisational compliance with Public Sector Equality Duty (PSED) from the Equality Act 2010.

All public sector bodies in England must demonstrate progress in eliminating racism (among other inequalities), promoting good relations and advancing equality.

Figure 3.2 shows the lack of diversity in senior pay bands in NHS trusts.

Since the launch of the WRES, there has been minimal, inconsistent progress toward improving the experiences of people of colour in the NHS (Box 3.12).

to *produce* the data, there is no mandate to *improve* the data and develop action plans to make lasting changes.

A benefit of WRES is that it has given ethnic minority personnel permission to speak about their experiences. It is no longer up to the individual to demonstrate the disparity – it can be shown across England for all ethnic minority employees. Some organisations have been more committed to addressing the disparity than others, contributing to regional (e.g. London) specific race equality plans.

Source: NHS Workforce Race Equality Standard (WRES), NHS England, 2021.

Box 3.12 Workforce Race Equality Standard (WRES) outcomes.

The 2021 WRES report showed that BME staff are 1.16 more likely to enter formal disciplinary processes than White staff, less likely to be appointed to posts from shortlisting, and more likely to be harassed and bullied by service users and managers.

However, the WRES has succeeded in shining a light on inequity in pay band distribution by race. The data have been used to call for interventions to build ethnic minority leadership pipelines, overhaul recruitment and incentivise organisations to include ethnic minorities in training opportunities. Unfortunately, apart from the mandate

Medical Workforce Race Equality Standard

The Medical Workforce Race Equality Standard (MWRES), led by NHS England, is an important step in measuring and driving fairness in medicine (Box 3.13). It supports equity measurement for all health workers in England through the NHS Workforce Race Equality Standard [18]. Pressing issues for medical personnel are postgraduate training, revalidation recommendations, differential attainment and fitness to practise complaints. All these areas require targeted action by professional bodies such as the General Medical Council (GMC) and medical educational establishments.

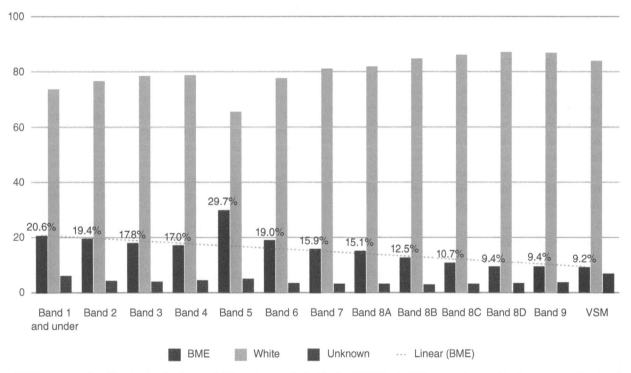

Figure 3.2 Percentage of staff by Agenda for Change (AfC) pay band and ethnicity for all NHS trusts. NHS pay bands are set by the government and go from band 1 to band 9 and do not include doctors or dentists. Most NHS workers are in bands 2–6. Cleaners, porters and healthcare assistants typically start in band 2, while newly qualified nurses, paramedics and midwives are in band 5. Bands 6 and above tend to have some level of management responsibility. Band 8 is split into multiple categories, with the highest paid being upper management. Band 9 is exclusively reserved for those in upper management. A nurse in band 8 may have a role such as a matron, which includes additional responsibilities such as workforce management, finance and budgeting, staff education and development, patient flow and performance management. The pay band after band 9 is for very senior management and is commanded by executives, board members and chairs in the NHS. Pay at this level is sometimes negotiated with employers or the government, depending on the position held.
Source: NHS Workforce Race Equality Standard (WRES), NHS England, https://www.england.nhs.uk/wp-content/uploads/2022/04/Workforce-Race-Equality-Standard-report-2021-.pdf 2021.

Box 3.13 **Medical Workforce Race Equality Standard.**

In 2020, the first Medical Workforce Race Equality Standard (MWRES) report was published to evaluate this workforce segment's experiences. It is the world's first to assess evidence of racism in healthcare faced by the national medical workforce.

Through the MWRES, England's health system can track whether collective efforts to tackle inequalities are working. For the most recent report, across all indicators, Black and minority ethnic (BME) doctors reported worse experiences at work compared to White doctors. Even when BME doctors become consultants, they continue to report greater levels of discrimination and harassment and feel less involved at work. The report also found that BME doctors are under-represented in senior positions, including consultant grade roles and academic positions. Of the 42% of BME doctors in the workforce, just 26% of clinical directors and 20% of medical directors are from BME heritage groups. There is also a significant pay gap, with White doctors earning 7% more than their BME colleagues.

Source: Medical Workforce Race Equality Standard (MWRES), NHS England, 2020.

The MWRES team is currently working to reduce the disproportionality of entry into local disciplinary processes and referrals to the GMC for ethnic minority and international medical graduate (IMG) doctors. It has suggested work to implement independent screening to support starting a formal local disciplinary process and referral to the GMC. This would be delivered by independent panels reviewing cases anonymously and making recommendations to the decision maker in each hospital. Other actions include standardising local arrangements for induction and ongoing support for IMG doctors and developing a process to diversify senior medical leadership appointments by improving the number of ethnic minority candidates in the shortlisting process.

Recruitment and retention are pressing problems for the health service in England. Without concerted efforts to improve the experiences of clinical staff (Box 3.14), the country is unlikely to be able to fulfil its duties of providing comprehensive healthcare to its population. Ongoing efforts to improve the experiences of the large cohort of BME clinical staff are a priority and have been recognised by recent government committee investigations [19].

Box 3.14 **Negative staff experiences.**

Research studies have consistently highlighted people of colour describing the experience of being bypassed for career development, requests for progression opportunities being blocked, and line managers failing to support their career aspirations. A survey by the BMA in 2022 showed that 76% of people said they had been subjected to at least one incident of racist behaviour, with 17% stating they experience it regularly. Of those who experienced racism, 71% chose not to report the incident either out of fear of being labelled a 'trouble-maker' or due to a lack of confidence that adequate action would be taken.

Below are some examples from studies by the King's Fund (2020), BMA (2022) and Sawley (2001).

'In our organisation currently, you know, Black staff are disproportionately disciplined ... we don't get access to training opportunities and promotions ... and we've got a couple of initiatives to try and change that, but it's still ...' she pauses, '... we've got a long way to go.'

'I've got people who are managing me who are racist ... My manager ... holds me back, stops me getting opportunities that [are given] to my White counterparts who ... [are] maybe not as experienced as me.'

'I think there's the feeling that sometimes you're not understood, or you're treated maybe a bit differently; not part of "in groups".'

'The managers above you are White, so again the role models are missing ... You don't see role models, any people of colour in higher positions, even within your own professional background.'

'One thing I find quite difficult is the more I speak up, the more my reputation becomes, "oh troublemaker" ... in organisations where relationships and reputation [are] everything you can easily get pushed out. You're just labelled difficult.'

Sources: The King's Fund (2020) Workforce Race Inequalities and Inclusion in NHS Providers. https://www.kingsfund.org.uk/publications/workforce-race-inequalities-inclusion-nhs
BMA (2022) Racism in medicine. www.bma.org.uk/media/5746/bma-racism-in-medicine-survey-report-15-june-2022.pdf
Sawley, L. (2001) Perceptions of racism in the health service. *Nursing Standard*, **15**(19), 33–35.

Conclusion

Racism occurs across healthcare in many parts of the world, affecting staff, patients, carers, researchers and other stakeholders. Racism in healthcare reproduces historical inequity that limits and reduces positive outcomes for those most affected. While research has relied on case studies and vignettes to explore and interrogate how racism impacts healthcare delivery and outcomes, there is still a lack of data-driven evidence that is robust, comparable and standardised to push for policy, strategy and process improvements. In some countries, such as Sweden, documenting race is considered to fuel inequality rather than limit it. Therefore, researchers seeking to make changes cannot work with quantifiable figures to put forward a case for change. This is similar in the UK, where different categories and inconsistent recording and documenting mechanisms make comparison across staff groups and healthcare areas problematic. In the UK, the government has issued a policy paper called 'Data saves lives: reshaping health and social care with data' [20]. More comprehensive research into patient experience has suggested interventions at micro and macro levels.

The micro level includes critical reflective practice, developing consciousness of race, racism and privilege and debiasing education, improving support for bystander interventions, improving forums for patients' lived experiences and using the outreach model to talk to communities reluctant to access services due to prior negative experience.

At a macro level, it requires collaborative work by professional bodies and educators to develop antiracist strategies to debias curricula. Healthcare providers should use robust equality impact analysis to interrogate processes and procedures. They should normalise race equity analysis in service development and planning and target recruitment, retention and progression interventions to address disparities between staff across different race groups [21].

Racism in healthcare is substantial. Investment in expanded research is required, especially in light of increased reliance on digital medicine and investment in technology (e.g. artificial intelligence) that relies on current data sources which lack diversity and inclusive methodology. The political will to address racism in healthcare is shifting, driven by the momentum of visible disparity in COVID-19 deaths and media coverage. In November 2021, the Secretary of State for Health and Social Care in the UK launched a review into potential racial bias in medical equipment to identify systematic inequalities in medical devices registered for use in the UK and to make recommendations on how these disparities can be rectified, and to consider what systems need to be in place to ensure emerging technologies are developed without perpetuating race inequality.

Further reading/resources

Ahlberg, B.M., Hamed, S., Bradby, H., Moberg, C. and Thapar-Björkert, S. (2022) 'Just Throw It Behind You and Just Keep Going': emotional labor when ethnic minority healthcare staff encounter racism in healthcare. *Frontiers in Sociology*. www.frontiersin.org/articles/10.3389/fsoc.2021.741202 (accessed 4 October 2022)

All-Party Parliamentary Group (APPG) (2021). No one's listening: an inquiry into the avoidable deaths and failures of care for sickle cell patients in secondary care. www.sicklecellsociety.org/wp-content/uploads/2021/11/No-Ones-Listening-PDF-Final.pdf (accessed 1 July 2022)

Alsan, M., Garrick, O. and Graziani, G. (2019). Does diversity matter for health? Experimental evidence from Oakland. *American Economic Review*, **109** (12), 4071–4111.

Baker, C. (2021) *NHS Staff from Overseas: Statistics*. House of Commons.

BMA (2021) COVID-19: analysing the impact of coronavirus on doctors. www.bma.org.uk/advice-and-support/covid-19/what-the-bma-is-doing/covid-19-analysing-the-impact-of-coronavirus-on-doctors (accessed 4 October 2022)

BMA (2022) Racism in medicine. www.bma.org.uk/media/5746/bma-racism-in-medicine-survey-report-15-june-2022.pdf (accessed 4 October 2022)

Cabinet Office Race Disparity Unit. www.gov.uk/government/organisations/race-disparity-unit (accessed 1 July 2022)

Care Quality Commission (CQC) (2022) Ethnic minority-led GP practices: impact and experience of CQC regulation. www.cqc.org.uk/publications/themed-work/ethnic-minority-led-gp-practices-impact-experience-cqc-regulation (accessed 1 June 2022)

Cortis, J.D. (2000) Perceptions and experiences with nursing care: a study of Pakistani (Urdu) communities in the United Kingdom. *Journal of Transcultural Nursing*, **11** (2) 111–118.

Cortis, J.D. (2004) Meeting the needs of minority ethnic patients. *Journal of Advanced Nursing*, **48** (1), 51–58.

Department of Health and Social Care (2017) Safer maternity care: progress and next steps. https://assets.publishing.service.gov.uk/government/uploads/system/uploads/attachment_data/file/662969/Safer_maternity_care_-_progress_and_next_steps.pdf (accessed 1 July 2022)

Fazil, Q. (2018) *Cancer and Black and Minority Ethnic Communities*. Race Equality Foundation

Hoffman, K.M., Trawalter, S., Axt, J.R. and Oliver, M.N. (2016) Racial bias in pain assessment and treatment recommendations, and false beliefs about biological differences between blacks and whites. *Proceedings of the National Academy of Sciences*, **113** (16), 4296–4301.

Joint Committee on Human Rights (2021) Black people, racism, and human rights: Government Response to the Committee's Eleventh Report of Session 2019–21. https://committees.parliament.uk/work/409/black-people-racism-and-human-rights/publications/

Kursumovic, E., Lennane, S. and Cook, T.M. (2020) Deaths in healthcare workers due to COVID-19: the need for robust data and analysis. *Anaesthesia*, **75** (8), 989–992.

Lammy, D. (2017) Lammy review: final report. www.gov.uk/government/publications/lammy-review-final-report (accessed 1 July 2022)

Macpherson, W. (1999) The Stephen Lawrence inquiry. https://assets.publishing.service.gov.uk/government/uploads/system/uploads/attachment_data/file/277111/4262.pdf (accessed 1 July 2022)

Public Health England (2020) *Disparities in the Risk and Outcomes of COVID-19*. London: PHE.

Ross, S., Jabbal, J., Chauhan, K., Maguire, D. and Randhawa M. (2020) Workforce race inequalities and inclusion in NHS providers. www.kingsfund.org.uk/publications/workforce-race-inequalities-inclusion-nhs (accessed 1 July 2022)

Sato, S. (2017) 'Operation Legacy': Britain's destruction and concealment of colonial records worldwide. *Journal of Imperial and Commonwealth History*, **45** (4), 697–719.

Schiebinger, L. (2017) *Secret Cures of Slaves: People, Plants, and Medicine in the Eighteenth-Century Atlantic World*. Stanford, CA: Stanford University Press.

Sawley, L. (2001) Perceptions of racism in the health service. *Nursing Standard*, **15** (19), 33–35.

Smedley, B.D., Stith, A.Y. and Nelson, A.R. (2003) *Unequal Treatment: Confronting Racial and Ethnic Disparities in Health Care*. Washington DC:, National Academies Press.

References

1 Williams, D.R. and Mohammed, S.A. (2009) Discrimination and racial disparities in health: evidence and needed research. *Journal of Behavior Medicine*, **32** (1), 20–47.

2 European Union Agency for Fundamental Rights (2011) Multiple discrimination in healthcare. https://fra.europa.eu/en/project/2011/multiple-discrimination-healthcare

3 Williams, E., Buck, D., Babalola, G. and Maguire, D. (2022) The King's Fund: what are health inequalities? www.kingsfund.org.uk/publications/what-are-health-inequalities.

4 Kapadia, D., Zhang, J., Salway, S., et al. (2022) Ethnic inequalities in healthcare: a rapid evidence review. www.nhsrho.org/publications/ethnic-inequalities-in-healthcare-a-rapid-evidence-review

5 Adas, M. (2008) *Colonialism and Science* (ed. H. Selin). Dordrecht: Springer Netherlands.

6 Arnold, D. (2000) *Science, Technology and Medicine in Colonial India*. Cambridge: Cambridge University Press.

7 Roy, R.D. (2017) *Malarial Subjects: Empire, Medicine and Nonhumans in British India, 1820–1909*. Cambridge (UK): Cambridge University Press.

8 Xiang, S. (2021) The persistence of scientific racism: Ernst Cassirer on the myth of race. *Critical Philosophy of Race*, **9** (1), 126–150.

9 Trawalter, S. and Hoffman, K.M. (2015) Got pain? Racial bias in perceptions of pain. *Social and Personality Psychology Compass*, **9** (3), 146–157.

10 Braun, L. (2021) Race correction and spirometry: why history matters. *Chest*, **159** (4), 1670–1675.

11 Williams, M.S., Myers, A.K., Finuf, K.D. et al. (2022) Black physicians' experiences with anti-black racism in healthcare systems explored through an attraction-selection-attrition lens. *Journal of Business and Psychology*, June 10, 1–14.

12 National Institute for Health Research (NIHR) (2020–21) Diversity data report 2020–21. www.nihr.ac.uk/about-us/our-key-priorities/equality-diversity-and-inclusion/NIHR-Diversity-Data-Report-2021.pdf.

13 Gower, M. (2022) Windrush generation: Government action to 'right the wrongs'. https://commonslibrary.parliament.uk/research-briefings/cbp-8779

14 Weekes-Bernard, D. (2013) *Nurturing the Nation – The Asian Contribution to the NHS since 1948*. London: Runnymede Trust.

15 Kingma, M. (2007) Nurses on the move: a global overview. *Health Service Research*, **42** (3 Pt 2), 1281–1298.

16 World Health Organization (2021) WHO global code of practice on the international recruitment of health personnel. www.who.int/publications/m/item/nri-2021.

17 Simpson, J.M. (2018) *Migrant Architects of the NHS: South Asian Doctors and the Reinvention of British General Practice*. Manchester: Manchester University Press.

18 NHS England (2021) *Medical Workforce Race Equality Standard (MWRES) WRES indicators for the medical workforce 2020*. London: NHS England.

19 Health and Social Care Committee (2022) Workforce: recruitment, training and retention in health and social care. https://committees.parliament.uk/publications/23246/documents/171671/default.

20 Department of Health and Social Care (2022). Data saves lives: reshaping health and social care with data. www.gov.uk/government/publications/data-saves-lives-reshaping-health-and-social-care-with-data/data-saves-lives-reshaping-health-and-social-care-with-data

21 Baker, C. (2021). *NHS Staff from Overseas: Statistics*. House of Commons.

CHAPTER 4

Ethnicity and Disease

Mohammad Rizwan Ali[1], Shehla Imtiaz-Umer[2], and John Frain[3]

[1] Fellow in Epidemiology, Department of Cardiovascular Sciences, College of Life Sciences, University of Leicester, Leicester, UK

[2] Equality, Diversity and Inclusion (EDI) Director, General Practice Task Force (GPTF) Derbyshire, UK; General Practitioner, UK; GMC Associate, UK

[3] General Practitioner, Clinical Associate Professor and Director of Clinical Skills, Division of Medical Sciences and Graduate Entry Medicine, University of Nottingham, Nottinghamm, UK

OVERVIEW

- Census data indicate that the diversity of the United Kingdom population is increasing each decade.
- Migrants are in better health when they emigrate to countries but over time their health can deteriorate because of their living conditions.
- Classifying people by the colour of their skin leads to discrimination which includes those in need of healthcare.
- Diseases in ethnic minority communities arise not only because of genetic risk but because of the wider determinants of health.
- Accurate recording and reporting of ethnicity are vital to identify and remedy health inequalities experienced by ethnic minority groups.

Introduction

The misuse of racial and ethnic categories in healthcare to stratify patients poses a significant risk of harm to them. The classification of ethnicity and race has a unique history in major Western countries. In the United States (US), racial categories were motivated by politics and racism. The House of Delegates classified every Black person in the US as three-fifths of a person to ensure the dominance of the southern states. Consequently, the first US Census in 1790 created three racial categories: White and Native people, each counted as one whole tax-paying person, and enslaved and Black people, counted as three-fifths. Although the legalisation was repealed in 1890, the segregation and marginalization of Black people continues in the US. In the United Kingdom, ethnicity data were first collected in 1976 for the National Dwelling and Household Survey. In 1991, England and Wales captured ethnicity data for the first time, reflecting the increasing population diversity (Table 4.1). The categorisation of individuals by skin colour has since enabled healthcare providers to identify discrimination in healthcare provision.

A global economy facilitates migration for many people worldwide. Often it is assumed that migrants are in poor health and will be a burden on services, including health. This is unsupported by the evidence (Box 4.1).

Table 4.1 Changing population diversity in England and Wales (2011 and 2021 Census Data).

Ethnicity	2011	2021
Asian		
Bangladeshi	0.8%	1.1%
Chinese	0.7%	0.7%
Indian	2.5%	3.1%
Pakistani	2.0%	2.7%
Asian other	1.5%	1.6%
Black		
Black African	1.8%	2.5%
Black Caribbean	1.1%	1.0%
Black other	0.5%	0.5%
Mixed		
Mixed White/Asian	0.6%	0.8%
Mixed White/Black African	0.3%	0.4%
Mixed White/Black Caribbean	0.8%	0.9%
Mixed other	0.5%	0.8%
White		
White: English, Welsh, Scottish, Northern Irish or British	80.5%	74.4%
White: Irish	0.9%	0.9%
White: Gypsy/Traveller	0.1%	0.1%
White: Roma	-	0.2%
White: Other	4.4%	6.2%
Other		
Arab	0.4%	0.6%
Any other	0.6%	1.6%

Source: https://www.ons.gov.uk/peoplepopulationandcommunity/culturalidentity/ethnicity/bulletins/ethnicgroupenglandandwales/census2021

This table shows the population change from 2011 until 2021 showing that the White British population proportion has decreased and most other ethnicities have increased during the same time period.

ABC of Equality, Diversity and Inclusion in Healthcare, First Edition. Edited by Shehla Imtiaz-Umer and John Frain.
© 2023 John Wiley & Sons Ltd. Published 2023 by John Wiley & Sons Ltd.

Box 4.1 **The 'healthy migrant' hypothesis.**

Migrants are a healthy group who self-select for migration, benefit from and succeed in migration. There is a lower prevalence of some conditions in ethnic minorities in the UK. Examples include cancers (lung and breast), anxiety, depression and suicide, peripheral vascular disease and alcoholism. This effect is also observed in Canada, United States and Australia.

Over time, the effect wanes. Migrants and ethnic communities face poor living conditions, more precarious employment with more significant occupational health risks, discrimination, poor social support and access to services, including health.

Previous studies have shown that foreign-born migrants tend to be healthier than non-migrants, known as the 'healthy migrant' effect. This is because migrants tend to skew to younger and healthier people than those who choose not to migrate. It is important to note that migrants are not a homogeneous group. Those migrating due to war or persecution because of protected characteristics have worse outcomes than those born in the UK and better outcomes for people who have migrated for employment, family or educational reasons. Overall, migrants are healthier than UK-born populations with a lower burden on public services such as the NHS (see Chapter 9).

The 'healthy migrant' hypothesis suggests migrant communities do not bring poor health with them but acquire risk from the host countries they live in. Established communities do show more adverse health outcomes (Figure 4.1). However, ethnicity is not causative of disease. Rather, it is associated with poorer health outcomes due to the social conditions in which the communities live and the discrimination towards them. A discussion of ethnicity and health must include consideration of the social determinants of disease (Figure 4.2).

Defining race and ethnicity

Literature regarding 'race' and 'ethnicity' is discordant. Often used interchangeably in medical literature and clinical practice, the terms can confuse healthcare professionals. These terms have been explained as social constructs and linked to biological characteristics. They have been used to both support and oppose the view that these terms have a biological basis.

To clarify, ethnicity captures the shared values and cultural norms of a group of people, whereas race is how individuals may identify themselves based on their physical appearance. Crucially, traits often associated with race, such as skin colour, bone density and craniofacial measurements, do not correlate with socially defined racial categories [1]. Both race and ethnicity are either socially or self-ascribed. It is now widely accepted that race and ethnicity are not biological classifications [2].

It is essential to clarify the distinction between race and ethnicity and their relationship to biology (Box 4.2). Although population-level similarities of people of a certain race may exist for a particular disease, this does not often apply at the individual level. Furthermore, as race and ethnicity are individuals or groups which are self-ascribing, mixed ethnicity can lead to further confusion when linking outcomes and analysing patient data. For example, a female of Pakistani and Caucasian heritage may identify as Pakistani, Caucasian or mixed. In medical databases, individuals may even be classified as one, two or all three of those listed previously.

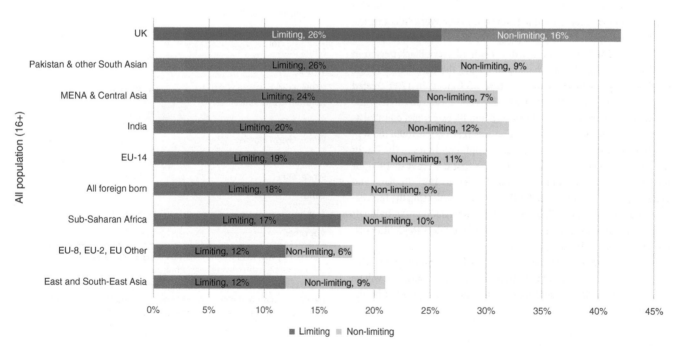

Population with limiting and non-limiting health problems by country of birth and age, 2019

Figure 4.1 Health in migrants vs non-migrants in the UK. A health condition is considered limiting if it reduces the person's ability to perform their usual day-to-day activities. This chart shows that those born in the UK have the highest proportion of limiting and non-limiting diseases compared to those that are not born in the UK.
Source: Adapted from Reino, M.R. The health of migrants in the UK. https://migrationobservatory.ox.ac.uk/resources/briefings/the-health-of-migrants-in-the-uk.

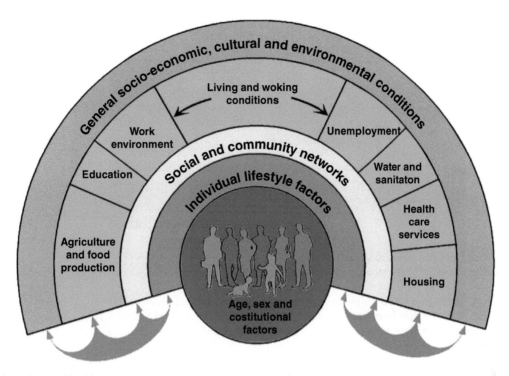

Figure 4.2 Social determinants of health.
Source: Adapted from Dahlgren, G. and Whitehead, M. (1991) *Policies and Strategies to Promote Social Equity in Health.* Stockholm, Sweden: Institute for Futures Studies.

> **Box 4.2 Descriptors of race and ethnicity.**
>
> *Race* – a group sharing some outward physical characteristics and some commonalities of culture and history.
>
> *Ethnicity* – a group of individuals linked through a combination of social practices, including history, language, religion, dress, food, music and ceremonial occasions linked to birth, marriage and death.
>
> *Nationality* – the legal identity conferred to individuals born in a particular country.
>
> *Genetic ancestry* – ancestors are the individuals you are biologically descended from, and ancestry is information about them and their genetic relationship to you.

Consequently, care must be taken when declaring increased incidence or prevalence of diseases or making inferences about an ethnic minority group. However, this does not mean these data should not be used in clinical care or research settings. It is crucial to identify these groups to compare illness prevalence and causes of inequalities to understand factors leading to worse outcomes across communities.

Ethnicity and discrimination in health

Many examples exist of ethnicity engendering bias towards ethnic minorities in healthcare. A patient may be identified by race or ethnicity when this has little relevance to their current condition in clinical practice. For example, when presenting patient histories, race, age and disease presentation are often discussed at the outset of case presentation. This reinforces the mistaken belief that race and ethnicity have a biological basis [3] (Box 4.3). The misinterpretation of biology with race has led to incorrect health and disease associations. A particularly egregious example is medical literature incorrectly perpetuating the association of pathologies with race [4] (Table 4.2).

Genetic factors in ethnic minorities

Genetic ancestry differentiates disease causation at the patient level (Box 4.2). Genetic ancestry is the general connection to people in the past. In a genetic context, ancestors are a person's biological antecedents [8]. Often, there are stark differences in outcomes for ethnic minority patients in epidemiological studies. These may be presented as a biological differentiation between

---

> **Box 4.3 Examples of ethnicity engendering bias towards ethnic communities.**
>
> *Dermatology*: skin colour has broad implications in medical practice as it is often wrongly associated with race. The current system for skin colour phototypes – the Fitzpatrick Classification of Skin Types scale – has explicit biases as there are Black, brown and White skin tones which have one, two and three types, respectively. This has led to biased artificial intelligence diagnostic algorithms [5]. Recently, the Monk Skin Tone Scale has been created to better represent skin tones of ethnic minorities.

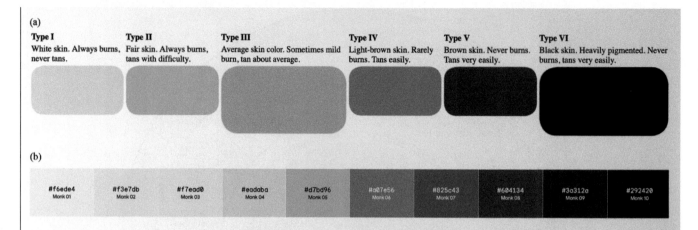

(a) Fitzpatrick Classification of Skin Types. (b) Monk Skin Tone Scale.

Source: 'Monk Skin Tone Scale' by Dr Ellis Monk, made available by Google LLC under the Creative Commons Attribution 4.0 international licence.

AI algorithms: machine learning and artificial intelligence (AI) are terms used for advanced statistical techniques to identify patterns in large datasets. Healthcare's adoption of patient-facing and clinical apps, which can diagnose and prognosticate, is rapidly increasing. However, there is potential for widening disparities for ethnic minorities. Often, AI data are from a homogeneous patient population (excluding minorities from data collection), complicating the broader generalisability of these algorithms [6].

Pulse oximetry: pulse oximetry has been used for decades to non-invasively measure heart rate and oxygen saturation using beams of light passing through skin and blood, which are modified by skin pigmentation. During the COVID-19 pandemic, inequalities were identified as pigmented skin patients were more likely to have falsely higher values of oxygen saturation than those with less pigment when compared to arterial blood gas results [7].

Table 4.2 Diseases traditionally associated with a patient's ethnicity.

System	Disease	Evidence supporting ethnic differences	Unsupported associations to ethnic differences	Contradictory to the evidence ethnicity is linked to disease
Deficiency disorders	Vitamin D	✕		
	Primary immunodeficiencies (IgA deficiency)		✕	
	Lactase (disaccharidase) deficiency		✕	
	Pernicious anaemia		✕	
Cancer	Squamous cell carcinoma			✕
	Breast cancer (incidence and epidemiology)	✕		
	Cancer incidence		✕	
	Lymphoid neoplasms	✕	✕	
	Tumours (testicular and prostate)		✕	
	Ewing sarcoma		✕	
	Malignant tumours of liver and biliary tract			✕
	Pancreatic tumour		✕	
Cardiac	Hypertensive vascular disease	✕		
Endocrinology	Diabetes mellitus and associated clinical features, e.g. diabetic nephropathy	✕		
Renal	Nephrotic syndromes		✕	
	Autosomal dominant polycystic kidney disease		✕	
	Benign nephrosclerosis	✕		

Table 4.2 (Continued)

System	Disease	Evidence supporting ethnic differences	Unsupported associations to ethnic differences	Contradictory to the evidence ethnicity is linked to disease
	Malignant hypertension and accelerated nephrosclerosis			×
Respiratory	Emphysema		×	
Gastric	*Helicobacter pylori* gastritis	×		
	Alcoholic liver disease (cirrhosis rates)		×	
Systemic disorders	Hypersensitive and autoimmune conditions, e.g. systemic lupus erythematosus	×		
	Systemic sclerosis (scleroderma)	×		
	Sarcoidosis	×		
Musculoskeletal	Osteoporosis		×	
Non-body system related	Infant mortality rate		×	

Evidence supporting ethnic differences: this column shows that there is evidence supporting the argument that ethnic differences in the disease exist.
Unsupported associations to ethnic differences: this column demonstrates that unsubstantiated claims were made between ethnicity and disease.
Contradictory to the evidence ethnicity is linked to disease: this column shows where the evidence is contradicted by the claims of a relationship between ethnicity and disease.
Whilst there is evidence of some diseases being linked to ethnicity, there are multiple examples of poorly evidenced disease associations to ethnicities. For example, it is clear to see that diseases such as pernicious anaemia, pancreatic tumours and osteoporosis have incorrectly been attributed to having a link with ethnicity.

races or not explained to the reader [9]. Genetic ancestry may provide a better marker of differentiation between patients. Although genetic data are not yet used in routine clinical practice, it would allow one to distinguish diseases caused by biological inheritance from immediate family members rather than the wider determinants of disease.

Diversity and inclusion within genetic databases are limited as most published literature has focused on the European ancestry population. In recent years, the overall proportion of European ancestry data has decreased because of the increased number of studies of East Asian populations and not an increase in the proportion of wider representation of ethnic minorities. This lack of diversity within datasets poses a significant challenge when using ancestral data to relate to the wider population, including ethnic minorities. A key example is the misclassification of African or unspecified ancestry because of a lack of diversity within the genetic research databases, which meant benign genetic variants were incorrectly categorised as pathogenic [10].

Evidence of ethnicity being deleterious for health outcomes

Genetic factors in ethnic minorities indicate an increased risk of disease. Genome-wide association studies (Box 4.4) have shown that Black men have an increased risk of developing prostate cancer because of the increased prevalence of genetic variants that are more common in Black men compared to Caucasian men. In addition, it is widely accepted that carriers of haemoglobin disorders, including thalassaemia and sickle cell disease, are more prevalent in people with African ancestry [11]. There are other advantages to using genetic data for ethnic minority groups. Treatments for disease are often tested against placebos in populations in randomised clinical trials (RCTs). The data from these studies are used to influence guidelines and policy recommendations for these treatments. However, RCTs have been known to recruit ethnic minorities poorly. This often plays out in the 'real world' as treatments may be rendered ineffective in ethnic minorities. For example, a common antiplatelet treatment has been shown to work poorly in Asians and Pacific Islanders because of the lack of genetic polymorphism that adequately metabolises the drug into its active constituent [12]. This lack of efficacy would probably have been identified if there had been sufficient people from minority groups in these trials.

Box 4.4 **Genome-wide association studies.**

With the completion of the Human Genome Project and the International HapMap project, research tools are available to identify genetic contributors to disease. Using the complete sets of DNA of large amounts of people, it is possible to find genetic variations which allow researchers to identify genetic associations with diseases. This technique is beneficial in common, complex disease analyses such as diabetes, cancer and cardiovascular disease. There are archives of data from genome-wide association studies, which can be accessed online via the Database of Genotype and Phenotype (dbGaP).

Wider determinants of disease in ethnic minorities

There are widely reported health inequalities for ethnic minorities within the UK [13] and USA [14,15]. Diseases such as diabetes and heart disease are often interpreted as being caused by ethnicity. Although genetic risk plays a crucial role in determining disease, environment often contributes to the risk of developing disease. These diverse environmental factors which impact health are known as social or wider determinants of health. Therefore, it is worth considering what the role of wider health determinants is for continued health inequalities. These social, economic and environmental factors include poor access to health, unemployment, multigenerational living and poor housing, which are the lived experiences of ethnic minorities and commonly associated with poorer health and outcomes. Evidence in the USA and the UK shows the differences in life expectancy between ethnicities (Tables 4.3 and 4.4). The Marmot Review 2010 raised awareness of the social (wider) determinants of health, emphasising how they affected health outcomes (see Further resources).

Wider determinants have a substantial role in causing health inequalities in ethnic minorities. A recent report by Public Health England, now known as the United Kingdom Health Security Agency (UKHSA), showed that ethnic minorities were at two times higher risk of mortality than White British people after accounting for confounding factors such as age, sex, area deprivation, income and education [16]. There are also overt examples of racism in the USA, such as redlining, contributing to a higher risk of adverse outcomes in ethnic minorities. Redlining is a legal form of residential segregation of ethnic minority communities which suffer disinvestment in education and social services, have high unemployment, poor access to health services and poor housing stock [9], perpetuating worse health outcomes.

Diseases associated with ethnicity are dogmatically and incorrectly discussed as being caused by biological and genetic factors without considering the wider determinants of health. Although the risk and prevalence may be higher in some cases for ethnic minorities, causation is multifactorial with a mix of genetic risk and environmental exposure. Examples of common diseases associated with ethnic minorities include hypertension, cardiovascular and renal disease risk in Black people; diabetes in South Asian people; and cardiovascular disease and renal failure in Roma people. Is disease prevalence higher in these groups because of genetic susceptibility or are structural inequalities causing this higher prevalence? It is essential to understand that disease prevalence is multifactorial in ethnic minority populations and also the wider population.

Considerable efforts are ongoing to highlight and remedy inequalities for ethnic minorities. There is the National Institute on Minority Health and Health Disparities in the US, while the Centre for Ethnic Health Research is working to reduce ethnic health inequalities in the UK. Furthermore, a landmark review published by the NHS Race and Health Observatory has highlighted ethnic health inequalities across specialties within healthcare in the UK (see Further resources).

Health outcomes and ethnicity

Conditions such as heart disease and diabetes are associated more with ethnic minorities (Box 4.5). Aside from disease prevalence, incidence and health outcomes have been shown to vary significantly across ethnic minorities compared to White ethnic groups.

> Box 4.5 **Cardiovascular disease (CVD) research of risk in ethnic minority groups.**
>
> Historically, some data had suggested that risk factors for cardiovascular disease varied by ethnicity. The INTERHEART study used a case–control design to quantify the risk factors for coronary heart disease worldwide [17]. The findings showed that nine risk factors

Table 4.3 Life expectancy at birth by sex and ethnic group: England and Wales 2011 to 2014.

Ethnic group	Females	Males	Sex gap (years)
Asian other	86.9	84.5	2.4
Bangladeshi	87.3	81.1	6.2
Black African	88.9	83.8	5.1
Black Caribbean	84.6	80.7	3.9
Black other	86.8	82.0	4.8
Indian	85.4	82.3	3.1
Mixed	83.1	79.3	3.8
Other	86.9	84.0	2.9
Pakistani	84.8	82.3	2.5
White	83.1	79.7	3.4
Ethnic group gap (years)	5.8	5.2	0.6

The data show the differential life expectancy for ethnic minority groups and White people. Whilst it shows the biggest differences between White females and Black African women and White men and Asian (other) men, it is essential to note that their health-related quality of life is unreported. A potential reason for the higher life expectancy found in the Black African and Asian Other ethnic groups is that these groups contain a higher proportion of more recent migrants than other ethnicities. Recent evidence has shown people who migrate tend to be healthier than others (Figure 4.1).

Office for National Statistics (ONS) figures based on the linkage of Census 2011 to Patient Register records and subsequent deaths followed up to 26th March 2014.

'Other' ethnic group includes Arab, Chinese and Other ethnic groups.

Source: www.ons.gov.uk/peoplepopulationandcommunity/birthsdeathsandmarriages/lifeexpectancies/articles/ethnicdifferencesinlifeexpectancyandmortality fromselectedcausesinenglandandwales/2011to2014

Table 4.4 Life expectancy at birth, by Hispanic origin, race, and sex: United States, 2006–2017.

Ethnic group	Females	Males	Sex gap (years)
Hispanic	84.3	79.1	5.2
Non-Hispanic Black	78.1	71.5	6.6
Non-Hispanic White	81	76.1	4.9
Ethnic group gap (years)	3.3	3.0	0.3

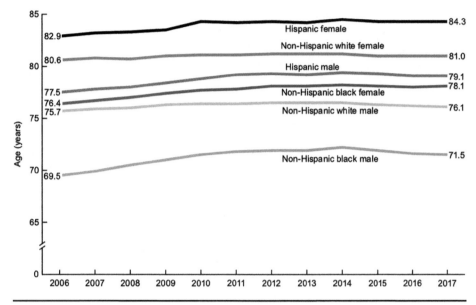

This table clearly shows that there is lower life expectancy for Black males in the USA compared to Hispanic and non-Hispanic males, with Hispanic females having the highest life expectancy compared to females of other ethnicities.

Source: www.cdc.gov/nchs/data/nvsr/nvsr68/nvsr68_07-508.pdf

accounted for 90% of an initial heart attack risk. Interestingly, the effect of these risk factors was consistent across ethnicities.

Research by Ho and colleagues [18] investigated the impact of differential exposure and susceptibility to CVD risk factors between different ethnic groups. Differential exposure is a higher level of prevalence of risk factors. For example, in South Asians, diabetes is a known risk factor for CVD and is more prevalent in South Asians than in other ethnicities.

Differential susceptibility is the risk factor that has a more substantial effect on ethnic minority groups. Specifically, a higher body mass index was more strongly associated with COVID-19 mortality for ethnic minorities than non-White ethnic groups during the initial waves of the COVID-19 pandemic in 2020. The findings showed that ethnic inequalities in CVD would be more effectively managed if interventions are tailored to particular ethnic groups based on need. For example, to reduce the excess risk of CVD, interventions to reduce socioeconomic deprivation in Black people and reduce diabetes incidence and prevalence in South Asians are needed.

COVID-19

Studies indicated that COVID-19 affected minority ethnic groups in the UK and the USA more than White populations, particularly in the first wave of the pandemic. Whilst subsequent waves showed a reduction in mortality differences, some ethnic minorities such as Bangladeshi and Pakistani groups (in the UK) continued to have a high risk of death. It was suggested that the increased risk was due to decreased health in ethnic minorities. However, further analysis showed that socioeconomic and structural factors played a role in the increased risk of death [19].

Diabetes

Type 2 diabetes mellitus (T2DM) is increasing in prevalence around the globe. In the UK, 6% of the population have a T2DM diagnosis and over 10% in the US. Diabetes incidence is disproportionately higher and has a 2–4 times higher prevalence in South Asians and Black ethnic groups than the White ethnic group. This is often attributed to genetic susceptibility in ethnic minorities but when genetic ancestry and socioeconomic deprivation are considered for developing T2DM in ethnic minorities, a recent study suggested that deprivation has a more significant causal effect on T2DM than genetic ancestry [20].

Renal disease

A particularly harmful myth that has been perpetuated in relation to renal disease has only recently been remedied in clinical guidelines (Box 4.6).

Box 4.6 **The myth of renal disease and ethnicity.**

Renal disease in minority ethnic populations, particularly Black people, exemplifies how racism can affect health outcomes. Creatinine is a by-product of exercise and is produced at a higher level in those exercising versus those who do not. It is also often raised in athletes compared to non-athletes. When testing Black people's renal function, elevated creatinine was common. Due to the prevailing misconception that Black people have superior muscle mass compared to other ethnicities, so-called 'correction factors' were created to normalise their creatinine levels, increasing the threshold before investigation/treatment was necessary. The myth of higher muscle mass in Black people and the need for adjustment markers of kidney function was perpetuated insidiously across the globe into routine clinical practice. This has led to stark inequalities in outcomes as Black people with chronic kidney disease were at higher risk of renal failure yet failed to meet the threshold for further investigation and treatment. Black people are now more likely to suffer from end-stage renal failure than their contemporaries. The National Institute for Health and Care Excellence (NICE) guidelines for chronic kidney disease were changed to remove creatinine adjustment for Black people in 2021.

Source: Kidney Research UK (2021) Ethnicity adjustment for kidney function testing removed from NICE chronic kidney disease guideline. Peterborough: Kidney Research UK.

Hypertension

There is significant variation in blood pressure (BP) between different ethnicities, with White adults having better BP control than other groups. Yet, differences in BP control within ethnic groups exist. The highest prevalence of hypertension is for Black people compared to other groups and a higher prevalence exists in South Asians compared to East/South-East Asian adults [21]. The mechanisms for these differences are poorly understood. It has been postulated that there may be molecular or biological processes but this requires further investigation. Multiple factors probably play a role in ethnic differences in hypertension, including genetic and social factors and risk stratification tools.

Strategies to improve ethnic minority healthcare outcomes

Whilst there is overwhelming evidence in the literature of widening inequalities for ethnic minorities, there are a few suggestions that improve health outcomes in ethnic minorities.

Coding in medical records

As ethnicity is often self-ascribed, recording these data accurately in the medical records is critical for identification and assessing outcomes in ethnic minority groups. Frequently, and especially in big

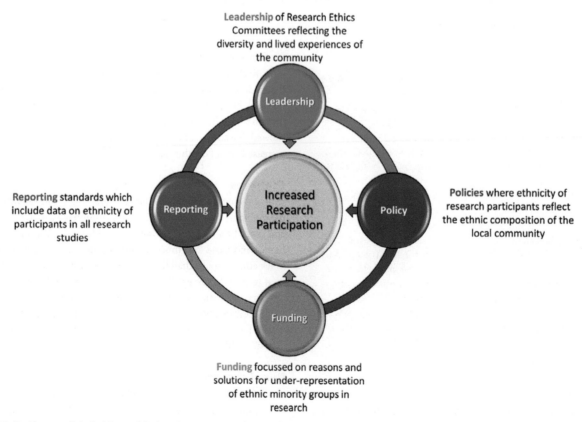

Figure 4.3 Health research inclusivity model. There is ongoing recognition of the lack of ethnic minority representation in health research. This model shows four pillars that are key to increasing research participation for ethnic minorities.
Source: Osuafor et al. [22], permission granted.

data cohorts such as the Clinical Practice Research Datalink (CPRD) in the UK, there can be records of multiple ethnicities for the same individual. Therefore, two steps are essential.

1 Ask the individual their ethnic information.
2 Accurately record this in their medical records.

Only when there is accurate, well-recorded and harmonised ethnicity data can we genuinely quantify, compare and understand the scope of the differences within ethnic minority groups and between ethnic minorities and the dominant population.

Risk stratification tools

Research shows significant differences between ethnic minorities and Caucasians. Identifying patients at higher risk earlier is becoming critical for efficient healthcare delivery and may improve outcomes for ethnic minorities. Whilst risk prediction algorithms used in the UK, such as QRISK (an algorithm which calculates an individual's 10-year risk of having a heart attack or stroke), incorporate ethnic differences, risk calculators in the US can be improved upon, with ongoing attempts being made to rectify this. However, this will only happen with increased coding of minority groups that is routinely and accurately completed.

Increased recruitment to clinical trials/cohorts

Research, and in particular clinical trials, identifies superior health interventions for patients. However, ethnic minorities are underrepresented in clinical trials. The exact extent is unknown as often clinical trials do not routinely record ethnicity data. Yet, there is evidence of significant differences in participation between White and ethnic minorities. Some steps can help remedy this. First, ethnicity must be recorded at the point of recruitment to a study and then reported in publications. Second, clinical trials are funded or sponsored by governmental agencies that have the power to mandate regulations within this arena. An example could be recruiting participants representing the local population where the research is taking place. To address this unmet need, a model of inclusivity in healthcare research is available (Figure 4.3).

Conclusion

We have addressed the critical terminology used when discussing ethnicity and race and considered the distinction between these terms and genetic ancestry. Although diseases have genetic risks associated with them, these exist within populations (including Caucasian) as well as between populations. It is therefore vital to consider the wider determinants of disease which play a significant role in understanding the ethnic inequalities existing in disease prevalence, incidence and outcomes. Societies with inherent structural racism impair the opportunities for living healthy lives for minority groups. Still, there is hope that these widening inequalities will be addressed in upcoming research and policy activities.

Further reading/resources

Kapadia, D. and Zhang, J. (2022) Ethnic inequalities in healthcare: a rapid evidence review. NHS Race Health Observatory. www.nhsrho.org/

wp-content/uploads/2022/02/RHO-Rapid-Review-Final-Report_v.7.pdf (accessed 26 October 2022)

Marmot, M. (2020) Health equity in England: the Marmot Review 10 years on. www.health.org.uk/publications/reports/the-marmot-review-10-years-on (accessed 1 July 2022)

NHS Race and Health Observatory (2022). Ethnic Inequalities in Healthcare: A Rapid Evidence Review. https://www.nhsrho.org/publications/ethnic-inequalities-in-healthcare-a-rapid-evidence-review/ (accessed 1 July 2022)

Raleigh, V. and Holmes, J. (2021) The the health of people from ethnic minority groups in England. www.kingsfund.org.uk/publications/health-people-ethnic-minority-groups-england (accessed 1 July 2022)

White, C. (2021) Ethnic differences in life expectancy and mortality from selected causes in England and Wales: 2011 to 2014. www.ons.gov.uk/peoplepopulationandcommunity/birthsdeathsandmarriages/life expectancies/articles/ethnicdifferencesinlifeexpectancyandmortality fromselectedcausesinenglandandwales/2011to2014 (accessed 1 July 2022)

References

1 Deyrup, A. and Graves, J.L. (2022) Racial biology and medical misconceptions. *New England Journal of Medicine*, **386** (6), 501–503.
2 Yudell, M., Roberts, D., DeSalle, R. and Tishkoff, S. (2016) SCIENCE AND SOCIETY. Taking race out of human genetics. *Science*, **351** (6273), 564–565.
3 Brett, A.S. and Goodman, C.W. (2021) First impressions – should we include race or ethnicity at the beginning of clinical case presentations? *New England Journal of Medicine*, **385** (27), 2497–2499.
4 Sheets, L., Johnson, J., Todd, T. et al. (2011) Unsupported labeling of race as a risk factor for certain diseases in a widely used medical textbook. *Academic Medicine*, **86** (10), 1300–1303.
5 Adamson, A.S. and Smith, A. (2018) Machine learning and health care disparities in dermatology. *JAMA Dermatology*, **154** (11), 1247–1248.
6 Jayakumar, S., Sounderajah, V., Normahani, P. et al. (2022) Quality assessment standards in artificial intelligence diagnostic accuracy systematic reviews: a meta-research study. *NPJ Digital Medicine*, **5** (1), 1–13.
7 Crooks, C.J., West, J., Morling, J.R. et al. (2022) Pulse oximeters' measurements vary across ethnic groups: an observational study in patients with Covid-19 infection. *European Respiratory Journal*, **59** (4), 2103246.
8 Mathieson, I. and Scally, A. (2020) What is ancestry? *PLoS Genetics*, **16** (3), e1008624.
9 Borrell, L.N., Elhawary, J.R., Fuentes-Afflick, E. et al. (2021) Race and genetic ancestry in medicine – a time for reckoning with racism. *New England Journal of Medicine*, **384** (5), 474–480.
10 Manrai, A.K., Funke, B.H., Rehm, H.L. et al. (2016) Genetic misdiagnoses and the potential for health disparities. *New England Journal of Medicine*, **375** (7), 655–665.
11 Modell, B. and Darlison, M. (2008) Global epidemiology of haemoglobin disorders and derived service indicators. *Bulletin of the World Health Organization*, **86** (6), 480–487.
12 Dean, L. (2018) Clopidogrel therapy and CYP2C19 genotype. www.ncbi.nlm.nih.gov/books/NBK84114.
13 Raleigh, V. and Holmes, J. (2021) The health of people from ethnic minority groups in England. www.kingsfund.org.uk/publications/health-people-ethnic-minority-groups-england.
14 National Academies of Sciences, Engineering and Medicine et al. (2017) The state of health disparities in the United States. In: *Communities in Action: Pathways to Health Equity*. Washington, DC: National Academies Press. www.ncbi.nlm.nih.gov/books/NBK425844
15 Fennelly, K. (2007) The 'healthy migrant' effect. *Minnesota Medicine*, **90** (3), 51–53.
16 Public Health England (2020) Disparities in the risk and outcomes of COVID-19. https://assets.publishing.service.gov.uk/government/uploads/

system/uploads/attachment_data/file/908434/Disparities_in_the_risk_and_outcomes_of_COVID_August_2020_update.pdf

17 Yusuf, S., Hawken, S., Ôunpuu, S. et al. (2004) Effect of potentially modifiable risk factors associated with myocardial infarction in 52 countries (the INTERHEART study): case-control study. *Lancet*, **364** (9438), 937–952.

18 Ho, F.K., Gray, S.R., Welsh, P. et al. (2022) Ethnic differences in cardiovascular risk: examining differential exposure and susceptibility to risk factors. *BMC Medicine*, **20** (1), 149.

19 Islam, N., Khunti, K., Dambha-Miller, H. et al. (2020) COVID-19 mortality: a complex interplay of sex, gender and ethnicity. *European Journal of Public Health*, **30** (5), 847–848.

20 Nagar, S.D., Nápoles, A.M., Jordan, I.K., and Mariño-Ramírez, L. (2021) Socioeconomic deprivation and genetic ancestry interact to modify type 2 diabetes ethnic disparities in the United Kingdom. www.thelancet.com/journals/eclinm/article/PIIS2589-5370(21)00240-6/fulltext

21 Fei, K., Rodriguez-Lopez, J.S., Ramos, M. et al. (2017) Racial and ethnic subgroup disparities in hypertension prevalence, New York City Health and Nutrition Examination Survey, 2013–2014. *Preventing Chronic Disease*, **14**: E33.

22 Osuafor, C.N., Golubic, R., and Ray, S. (2021) Ethnic inclusivity and preventative health research in addressing health inequalities and developing evidence base. www.thelancet.com/journals/eclinm/article/PIIS2589-5370(20)30416-8/fulltext.

CHAPTER 5

Representation in Healthcare Training

Diana Akpeki[1], Zunaira Dara[2], and John Frain[3]

[1] Final Year Graduate Entry Medical Student, University of Nottingham, Nottingham, UK
[2] Foundation Doctor, Greater Glasgow and Clyde, Scotland, UK
[3] General Practitioner and Clinical Associate Professor and Director of Clinical Skills, Division of Medical Sciences and Graduate Entry Medicine, University of Nottingham, Nottingham, UK

OVERVIEW

- Social role models and awareness of the possibility of aspiring to a role in higher-status professions are essential to fostering inclusive healthcare professions.
- Students feel excluded when they don't see themselves and their community reflected in the teaching content and presentation of healthcare training.
- Exclusion can foster feelings of imposter syndrome, common among healthcare students but particularly in those from minority groups.
- Proper representation in curricula of all communities encountered in clinical practice is an issue of human dignity and patient safety.
- Achieving improved representation across the curriculum is increased through listening to the student voice and understanding their needs.
- An inclusive curriculum will be reflected across the learning culture, content and assessment and will improve the competence of all students.

Introduction

Bias against the self (internalised bias, see Chapter 2) leads to reduced self-esteem, aspiration for one's own future achievements and acceptance of stereotypes about one's own community. Clark's 'Doll Test' demonstrated that these beliefs are established very early in life (Box 5.1). The culture of the educational environment, including visible role models, is crucial in supporting students in overcoming these feelings.

Box 5.1 **The Doll Test [1].**

The Doll Test [1].Drs Kenneth and Mamie Clark, psychologists, asked African-American children aged three to seven to identify the race of four dolls. The dolls were identical except for skin colour. The children were asked to express a preference for the colour of the dolls. Most children preferred the White doll and were likelier to attribute positive characteristics to it. Some children made negative remarks about the Black doll. The Clarks concluded that the still young African-American children's experience of discrimination had already produced in them feelings of inferiority and low self-esteem.

The Clarks' work contributed to the US Supreme Court's ruling in Brown v Board of Education 1954, that the segregation of public schools was unconstitutional. The order stated, 'To separate African-American children from others of similar age and qualifications solely because of their race generates a feeling of inferiority as to their status in the community that may affect their hearts and minds in a way unlikely ever to be undone'. Kenneth Clark believed segregation damaged not only African-American children but White children too.

On 25th June 2015, London became home to the 19th location of KidZania, an 'edutainment' children's theme park. Unlike other theme parks, it allows children to experience various career options within carefully thought-out intricate settings. KidZania's global education director, Dr Graus, has widely promoted this feature. According to Dr Graus, without social role models, visual representation and awareness, children cannot aspire to higher-status professions such as medicine [2]. The implications of this for healthcare are far wider than childhood aspiration and include staff recruitment, retention, wellbeing and patient safety.

Unfortunately, even after high achievers overcome limited career advice, low teacher expectations and financial constraints [3], they must learn to navigate unfamiliar higher education settings with few or no relatable role models (Box 5.2). Research has evidenced the severe impact of underrepresentation on individuals from minority backgrounds within the medical profession. They often feel excluded from social spheres, have experienced some form of bullying, and are more likely to face disciplinary actions and leave the profession altogether [4]. This adds to the pressures of an already intense course (Figure 5.1). Hence, efforts must be made to ensure that future healthcare professionals are genuinely welcomed, valued and included rather than the tokenistic approach often adopted by institutions.

Box 5.2 **'I just can't see myself in healthcare'.**

'I thought coming into a healthcare environment it would be a mind-broadening experience, that I'd learn about other people and

ABC of Equality, Diversity and Inclusion in Healthcare, First Edition. Edited by Shehla Imtiaz-Umer and John Frain.
© 2023 John Wiley & Sons Ltd. Published 2023 by John Wiley & Sons Ltd.

other cultures. Maybe even that I could teach others from my own experience. It's not been like that at all. I never see people like myself. All the case studies are about nice White people and families. The examination demonstrations are by young, White male athletic types. Where our simulation cases or role plays include ethnic minorities, they are very stereotypical, Asian taxi drivers or aggressive Black people. It's the same with family units. Everyone is heterosexual and able-bodied. There is no diversity. I know this upsets my LGBT friends as much as it does me. It just confirms the lack of belonging we always feel. If our future patients are all going to conform to the stereotypes, it would, perhaps, be understandable. We all know that won't be the case, though. So, all in all, I feel let down and that I am not being properly trained.'

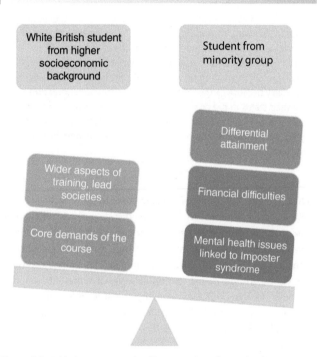

Figure 5.1 Added pressures on healthcare students from minority groups.

What do we mean by representation?

French social psychologist Serge Moscovici developed the concept of social representation in 1961. Figure 5.2 outlines Moscovici's definition of social representation and its two functions. Essentially, the purpose of social representation is 'to make something unfamiliar familiar' and 'enable achievement of a shared social reality' [5]. As Sammut and Howarth put it, social representations 'conventionalise objects, persons and events by placing them in a familiar context'. When established, 'they serve to influence social behaviour and social identities' [6].

Research has proposed social representations as systems of communication and social influence reflecting the social realities of different groups in society. Social representations shape how individuals view themselves and the world around them and how they fit into that world. For healthcare students, staff and patients, being unable to see themselves in how teaching is presented to them may lead to feelings of exclusion and being undervalued.

Why does representation matter?

When thinking of representation, it can be interesting to consider what images come to our minds when we think of a specific type of person based on their skills, experience or talents. To consider this in more depth, consider the reflective exercise in Figure 5.3.

Interactive discussion task:

- With your eyes closed, pause and visualise a harpist, a violinist or any classical musician.
- What do they look like to you?

Reflective exercise:

- Who came to your mind?
- Why do you think that was?
- What social identities would you associate with a classical musician?
- Try another occupation, e.g. sports person, actor, artist, etc.

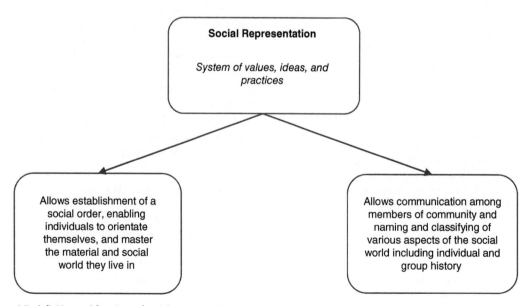

Figure 5.2 Moscovici's definition and functions of social representation.
Source: Adapted from Moscovici, S. (1961/1976) La Psychanalyse, Son Image et Son Public, 2nd edn. Paris: Presses Universitaires de France.

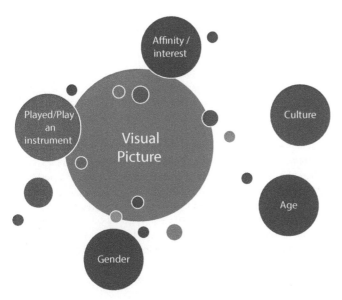

Figure 5.3 What do you see in your mind's eye?

A roadmap for diversity in medicine includes the following factors.

- Acknowledge, publicly, how our institutions have been complicit in and advantaged by the systematic discrimination of people of colour.
- Commit to investing at least 3% of our organisations' operating budget to support diversity, equity and inclusion.
- Cultivate the future supply of talented individuals from diverse backgrounds.
- Use restorative justice to optimise equity in the learning and work environment.
- Educate physicians to address the social determinants of health, including racism.
- Dedicate institutional resources to recruit and retain faculty historically underrepresented in medicine by race and ethnicity.

Source: Boatright, D., Berg, D. and Genao, I. (2021) A roadmap for diversity in medicine during the age of COVID-19 and George Floyd. *Journal of General Internal Medicine*, **36**(4), 1089–1091.

- What if you couldn't see yourself or someone like you in any of these scenarios?
- How does that make you feel?
- How does it feel for others who can't see themselves in these roles?

Your reflection will differ based on factors including age, cultural background, socioeconomic factors and prior exposure to classical music. However, anxiety may arise when a person from one background cannot imagine this could be someone who looks like them or imagines only persons with similar characteristics (e.g. a young, athletic White male).

Extrapolating from this exercise, consider the impact on healthcare staff, patients and organisations if they don't see themselves or their community presented in the content of their training. By omitting minority groups from visible representation in the healthcare curriculum, the implication is that healthcare is only for certain groups of people and that, as an ethnic or other minority individual, you have little value in the field of medicine. This is the reality for significant numbers of students arriving on day 1, with excitement and anticipation, to commence their healthcare training. Although there is evidence of prior action by medical schools in the UK (see Further resources), sadly, it took the death of George Floyd in 2020 and the resulting worldwide Black Lives Matter protests to galvanise action to urgently address the lack of representation of brown-skinned patients within medical education (Box 5.3).

Box 5.3 **Black Lives Matter and the legacy of George Floyd.**

The murder of George Floyd in May of 2020 and the clear racial disparities in COVID deaths throughout the pandemic led medical students and the wider medical community to call out racism within medicine. In the UK, a petition demanding better representation of Black, Asian and minority ethnic people in clinical teaching received over 200 000 signatures, leading to the formation of the UK Medical Schools Council Equality, Diversity and Inclusion Alliance in 2021.

Imposter syndrome

Imposter syndrome was first described by Clance and Imes in 1978 [7]. It was observed among high-achieving women and defined as an internal struggle that brings about feelings of inadequacy and chronic self-doubt. It can make the sufferer feel like a 'fraud', as though they do not deserve their success, despite evidence to the contrary. Imposter syndrome is associated with anxiety, depression and low self-esteem (Figure 5.4).

Imposter syndrome has been described as comprising four facets:

- anxiety
- self-doubt
- perfectionism
- fear of failure.

It is commonly assumed that imposter syndrome arises from one's own limitations or mental health issues. This 'blames the victim' and transfers the responsibility to the individual, overlooking or trivialising the role external factors, including institutional

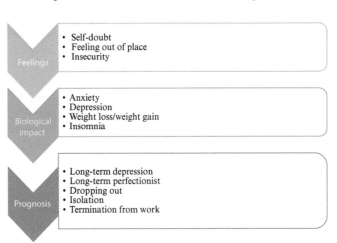

Figure 5.4 The impacts of imposter syndrome.

elements, play in the process. Imposter syndrome is not unique within the medical profession, nor only experienced by those who belong to minority groups. Depending on the screening method, up to 80% of those studying for a medical degree will experience this phenomenon at some point during their training or continue into their career post qualification [8]. This is because the medical profession is highly competitive and filled with high flyers who desire perfection. Figure 5.5 illustrates factors that contribute to imposter syndrome.

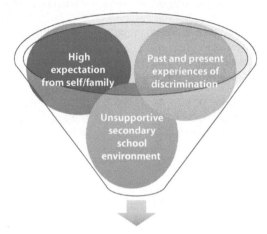

Feelings of inadequacy

Figure 5.5 Factors contributing to imposter syndrome.

Studies have shown that prevalence is higher among ethnic minority groups [9]. How ethnic minority students experience imposter syndrome differs from how White students experience it. Ethnic minority students may experience imposter syndrome with the added layers of daily microaggressions, discrimination and racism (see also Chapter 3). Feelings of imposter syndrome intersect with underrepresentation in teaching and content resource, bias and exclusion [10] (see also Chapter 11).

Intensified feelings of not belonging may be due to many unwelcoming experiences. It is unlikely a White British medical student would be asked 'Where are you really from?' during their training. These experiences of discrimination determine the manifestation of impostor syndrome among ethnic minority students and often result in burnout and depression [11].

Experiences of imposter syndrome are not identical across minority students. One American study reported that the impact of imposter feelings on depression was significantly higher in Black students compared to Asian or Latino students. Multiple studies have found that Black students report substantially higher perceived discrimination than any other ethnic minority group. McClain et al. found that stress factors within certain minority groups' status were predictors of mental health issues [12].

For ethnic minority students, imposter syndrome is a deeply complex issue that is not confined to their capabilities but also tied to their identities and whether there is a place for them in medicine. Imposter syndrome among minority students is detrimental to mental health, wellbeing and academic performance. It contributes to the differential attainment ('awarding gap') observed in minority students (Box 5.4).

Box 5.4 **Differential attainment among minority medical students (the 'awarding gap').**

Differences in academic attainment are observable across student groups when analysed for characteristics including age, gender and ethnicity. In medicine, this was first reported in 1995, when Manchester Medical School admitted that male students with Asian surnames were more likely to fail their clinical but not written exams. A systematic review confirmed widespread differences in academic performance for ethnic minority students across medical schools, different examination types and among undergraduates and postgraduates. The General Medical Council has produced guidance for medical schools on how to address this within curriculum design.

Differential attainment remained when factors including socioeconomic status, pre-university academic/non-academic achievement, study habits, first language, motivation for being a doctor and personality were considered. This also pertained when assessments were electronically marked to reduce examiner bias [13].

Sources: Dillner, L. (1995) Manchester tackles failure rate of Asian students. *BMJ*, **310**, 209.

Woolf, K., Potts, H.W. and McManus, I.C. (2011) Ethnicity and academic performance in UK trained doctors and medical students: systematic review and meta-analysis. *BMJ*, **342**, d901.

The culture of healthcare can leave staff, including medical students and doctors, feeling they must not display weakness or failure. There is a well-documented erosion of healthcare students' empathy, particularly upon entering the clinical years. Key domains influencing empathy include the following [14]:

- Course of studies: hands-on experience, role models, science and theory, teaching on importance of empathy.
- Students: insecurities, lack of routine, previous work experiences, mood, maturity, personal level of empathy.
- Patients: 'easy' and 'difficult' and their state of health.
- Environment: time pressure and stress, work and job dissatisfaction.

Hence when a student confides in their peers about sensitive racial experiences, issues of sexuality or disability, this often falls on unsympathetic ears. This is coupled with the inability of many individuals to fully grasp the reality of racial or other discrimination, especially when they do not belong to a minority group. Dismissive responses from peers may be interpreted as acceptance of the discrimination and a signal that the non-White or other minority student's more difficult medical training is insignificant or exaggerated. Subsequently, the non-White student is left still seeking validation, acceptance and belonging. The feeling is worsened depending on how dark one's skin is, with colourism contributing to a complex dynamic [15].

From entry until the later stages of a career, it can seem the student's existence is overshadowed by competition with peers and attitudes from staff constantly reminding them of their place [16]. Institutions openly publish student grades, ranking performance and ultimately heightening feelings of anxiety. Labels such as 'top deciles' and 'high educational performance' scores are widely sought to avoid the consequences of failure. There is the anxiety of less freedom to choose one's future specialty, training location and respect from colleagues. Peers may drift slowly from ally to rival. This fosters an unhealthy culture and a passive-aggressive environment. The aspiration of a compassionate, patient-centred, caring and empathic vocation is abandoned.

The experience of medical students from ethnic and other minority backgrounds is a less positive and supportive learning environment, as well as discrimination and racial harassment during medical school [17].

Addressing representation and inclusion in the curriculum

Despite 40% of medical students identifying as belonging to an ethnic minority group, medical school educators are often ill prepared to discuss ethnicity and broader systemic issues such as inequity and health inequalities affecting ethnic and other minority patients (e.g. LGBTQ+, disability, women's health). Often teaching around minority patients appears tokenistic and based on outmoded stereotypes. Cultural and other differences are presented as a hurdle to be overcome. This mentality needs to change. Britain is a diverse and multicultural society, and healthcare training needs to fully reflect this and the needs of all patients and healthcare staff.

Medical schools should provide students with opportunities to think about and reflect on this diversity, challenge their beliefs and biases, and have a safe space to ask difficult questions to increase their understanding of other cultures (Box 5.5). Cultural differences should not be presented as a burden to healthcare staff. There should be an emphasis on medical education being taught in a way that fosters understanding, compassion and respect and enables students to adapt their care sensitively (see Chapters 12 and 13). This approach is consistent with the values promoted by the GMC's *Good Medical Practice* (see Further resources).

Box 5.5 **Creating safe spaces for student discussion.**

All healthcare students should have the opportunity for safe discussion of representation and inclusion in healthcare. Real-life clinical scenarios can help facilitate this. Examples of sessions and content could include the following.

- Equality, diversity and inclusion in healthcare
  - Racial discrimination on clinical placement
  - Same-sex couples' experience of accessing healthcare
  - Racial discrimination in postgraduate assessment training
  - Experience of transgender medical students
  - Discrimination of females returning from maternity leave
  - Being an 'active bystander'
- Women in healthcare
  - Sexual harassment by colleagues
  - Boundaries between patients and healthcare staff
  - Sexism in medicine and choice of career path
  - Sexual harassment by a patient
  - Handling aggression and abusive behaviour
- Bias in medicine
  - Assessment of chest pain in women
  - Forms of bias in medicine
  - Implicit bias
  - Impact of bias on diagnostic accuracy
  - Racial bias in the assessment of pain

There are, of course, many more possible topics for discussion.

Where are we now?

Historically, medicine was an inaccessible career for women and non-White people (see Chapter 6). We have come a long way since then. As of 2017, the number of women entering medical school outnumbers men, with women accounting for 59% of admissions [18]. Currently, women make up 48% of UK-licensed doctors but it is no secret that women remain underrepresented in specific medical fields (e.g. surgery). Even in specialties with similar numbers of men and women (e.g. primary care), women are less likely to hold leadership positions (see Chapter 6). Similarly, for ethnic and other minority groups, representation in leadership roles is lower in practice and medical education (see Chapter 3). The adverse impact of the lack of minority representation in decision-making roles on minority ethnic communities has been well documented. Research has established that equality in healthcare outcomes, medical education and staff retention cannot be achieved without representation [19].

Changing the narrative

Institutions and teachers need to engage with the need for representation in healthcare both for ensuring adequate training and wellbeing for student and for the safety of all patients. The student voice is essential in identifying areas of need and how best to achieve this [20]. Teachers and institutions may worry about making mistakes and inadvertently causing offence. Acknowledging one's own need to learn and an approach of cultural humility is generally appreciated and received with understanding. Students are frequently helpful in providing advice on developing and piloting teaching resources. They can also advise on the use of appropriate terminology. The teacher's contribution to this collaborative approach is also helpful in modelling openness about knowledge gaps, teamworking and reflective practice, which are qualities required in tomorrow's health professionals.

Revealing 'hidden figures'

One consequence of the historical lack of representation in healthcare training is the invisibility of significant role models from minority backgrounds. In our own institution, we have begun to highlight a 'clinician of the week' (Box 5.6), individuals from an ethnic minority, LGBTQ+, disabled and women doctors who have made significant contributions to healthcare. In fact, these 'hidden figures' are not so difficult to find (see Further resources). Many academic and regulatory body websites now host pages providing details of historical and living figures who have overcome barriers to achievement. We can also highlight examples of former students now reaching positions of influence in their chosen specialties to our students.

Increasing visual representation

The individual as a patient and the individual as a clinician are essential aspects of representation. However, highlighting the modes of presentation of clinical signs in different skin tones is also important for patient safety and inclusion. It is a patient-centred activity to discuss how best to diagnose symptoms and physical signs in the context of the individual patient presenting with a health condition. In this respect, it is iterative and based on the needs of each individual patient living within their own unique context [20]. The image banks

Box 5.6 **Clinician of the week.**

A PowerPoint slide at the beginning of each clinical skills session highlights a clinician who has overcome barriers to achievement in medicine.

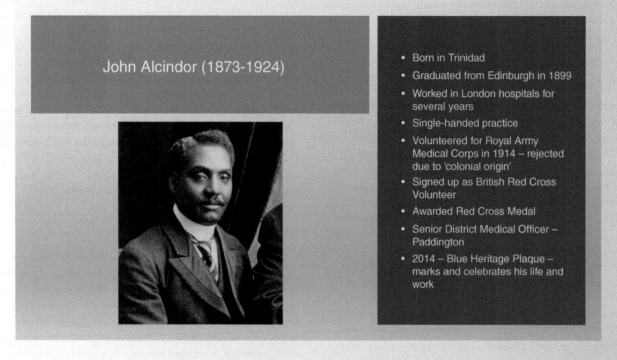

John Alcindor (1873-1924)

- Born in Trinidad
- Graduated from Edinburgh in 1899
- Worked in London hospitals for several years
- Single-handed practice
- Volunteered for Royal Army Medical Corps in 1914 – rejected due to 'colonial origin'
- Signed up as British Red Cross Volunteer
- Awarded Red Cross Medal
- Senior District Medical Officer – Paddington
- 2014 – Blue Heritage Plaque – marks and celebrates his life and work

'I had never seen positive examples of people who looked like me and came from a similar background, so compiling this list of people was incredibly vindicating for me.'

(Student feedback on 'Clinician of the week')

Source: Unknown author / Wikimedia Commons / Public domain

of resources such as Clinical Key (see Further resources) again provide a range of material. Medical student Malone Mukwende's 'Mind the Gap' handbook galvanised thinking about the importance of teaching the presentation of signs in Black and brown skin. It is an excellent resource to both facilitate discussion and address the diagnosis of skin conditions. In addition, institutions can develop a range of slide sets demonstrating clinical skills by professionals from all backgrounds, such as communication and physical examination skills, rather than the 'White male doctor' (Figure 5.6).

Course content

Although important, visual representation is insufficient. Course content needs also to reflect the healthcare needs of minority communities. These need to be woven into the substance of teaching content so it is patient centred and focused on the individual patient's healthcare needs rather than stereotypes regarding their particular identities. This may be the anxieties around accessing healthcare for an LGBTQ+ patient, chest pain in women or prostate cancer in a middle-aged Black man (see Further resources).

A range of changes across a curriculum centred on the needs of individual patients can be made to make the training and inclusion of all a step towards reality (Box 5.7). Ideally, once the possibility of

triggering additional assessment-induced anxiety is addressed, professional attitudes and clinical practice skills of inclusion in healthcare need to be included in the formative and summative assessment of every student's training.

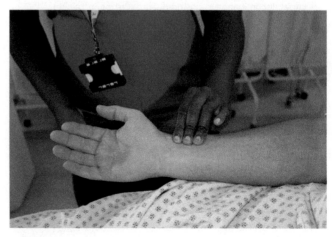

Figure 5.6 Individual as clinician: representation in the demonstration of physical examination skills.

Box 5.7 **Improving inclusion in a Clinical Skills curriculum.**

The following maps changes to inclusion in a preclinical Clinical Skills curriculum on the Graduate Entry Medicine (GEM) course at the University of Nottingham.
- Discussion workshops
  - Equality, diversity and inclusion in healthcare
  - Bias in medicine
  - Implicit bias
  - Women in healthcare
  - Sexual orientation and gender identity
- Clinical photos and video resources
  - Individual as patient (physical signs)
  - Individual as clinician (communication and examination)
- Course content
  - Reviewing the evidence base and literature
  - Inclusive clinical reasoning scenarios and vignettes
  - Inclusive history taking and role plays
  - Active bystander resources
- Staffing
  - Diversifying the patient actor group
  - Diversifying patient volunteers for bedside teaching and assessments (OSCEs)
- Simulation resources
  - Manikins with darker skin tones

Conclusion

We hope the reader will be inspired to broaden their understanding of the complex nature of equality, diversity and inclusivity. The suggested approaches can guide potential solutions and foster more in-depth discussions within healthcare courses. Beyond this, we aim to promote and preserve compassion amongst all physicians. For the ethnic and other minority students reading this text, we hope that some of the student experiences mentioned demonstrate that you are not alone and that the culture is changing. We are entering better times.

Further reading/resources

BMA (2022) Racial harassment charter for medical schools. www.bma.org.uk/advice-and-support/equality-and-diversity-guidance/race-equality-in-medicine/racial-harassment-charter-for-medical-schools (accessed 24th October 2022)

ISSUU (2022) Decolonising the curriculum toolkit. https://issuu.com/soyouwanttodecoloniseyourmedicalschool/docs/so_you_want_to_decolonise_your_medical_school_v2_ (accessed 24th October 2022)

General Medical Council (2022) Differential attainment project. www.gmc-uk.org/education/standards-guidance-and-curricula/projects/differential-attainment (accessed 24th October 2022)

General Medical Council (2022) Good Medical Practice. www.gmc-uk.org/ethical-guidance/ethical-guidance-for-doctors/good-medical-practice (accessed 24th October 2022)

Hidden Harms (2022) The Professional (Report). https://static1.squarespace.com/static/61c3bb8936cec959bee7a9c8/t/6283ddc4cefa022d95f81060/1652809185478/TheProWeb.pdf. (accessed 26th October 2022)

Hidden Harms. The Patient (Report). https://static1.squarespace.com/static/61c3bb8936cec959bee7a9c8/t/6283b21b49f55a172cd76c4c/1652798003194/HHThePatient.pdf (accessed 26th October 2022)

Kidzania. https://kidzania.co.uk (accessed 24th October 2022)

Linton, S. (2020) Taking the difference out of attainment. *BMJ*, **368**, m438.

Mind the gap – black and brown skin. www.blackandbrownskin.co.uk/mindthegap (accessed 24th October 2022)

Melanin Medics. www.melaninmedics.com (accessed 24th October 2022)

NHS Learning Academy – The Doll Test. https://learninghub.leadershipacademy.nhs.uk/guides/the-impact-of-stereotyping-clark-doll-test/steps/the-clark-doll-test-2 (accessed 24th October 2022)

Women in surgery. www.rcseng.ac.uk/careers-in-surgery/women-in-surgery (accessed 25th October 2022)

References

1 Legal Defense Fund. A revealing experiment: Brown v. Board of Education and 'The Doll Test'. www.naacpldf.org/brown-vs-board/significance-doll-test (accessed 16th October 2022)

2 Kidzania. https://kidzania.co.uk.

3 Universities UK and National Union of Students (2019) Black, asian and minority ethnic student attainment at UK universities: #closing the gap. www.universitiesuk.ac.uk/sites/default/files/field/downloads/2021-07/bame-student-attainment.pdf (accessed 16th October 2022)

4 BMA (2022) Racism in medicine. www.bma.org.uk/media/5746/bma-racism-in-medicine-survey-report-15-june-2022.pdf (accessed 16th October 2022)

5 Moscovici, S. (1984) The phenomenon of social representations. In: *Social Representations* (eds R. Farr and S. Moscovici), 3–69. Cambridge: Cambridge University Press.

6 Sammut. G. and Howarth, C. (2014) Social representations. In: *Encyclopedia of Critical Psychology* (ed. T. Teo). New York: Springer.

7 Clance, P.R. and Imes, S.A. (1978) The imposter phenomenon in high achieving women: dynamics and therapeutic intervention. *Psychotherapy: Theory Research and Practice*, **15** (3), 241–247.

8 Bravata, D.M., Watts, S.A., Keefer, A.L. (2020) Prevalence, predictors, and treatment of impostor syndrome: a systematic review. *Journal of General Internal Medicine*, **35** (4), 1252–1275.

9 Gallegos, M., Gonzales, D., and Shah, P. (2020) Imposter syndrome among minority medical students. www.acponline.org/membership/medical-students/acp-impact/archive/august-2020/imposter-syndrome-among-minority-medical-students (accessed 17th October 2022)

10 Khan, M. (2021) Imposter syndrome – a particular problem for medical students. *BMJ*, **375**, n3048.

11 Dyrbye, L.N., Thomas, M.R. and Huschka, M.M. (2006) A multicenter study of burnout, depression, and quality of life in minority and nonminority US medical students. *Mayo Clinic Proceedings*, **81** (11), 1435–1442.

12 McClain, S., Beasley, S., Jones, B. et al. (2016) An examination of the impact of racial and ethnic identity, impostor feelings, and minority status stress on the mental health of black college students. *Journal of Multicultural Counseling and Development*, **44**, 101–117.

13 Woolf, K., McManus, I.C., Potts, H.W. and Dacre, J. (2013) The mediators of minority ethnic underperformance in final medical school examinations. *British Journal of Educational Psychology*, **83** (Pt 1), 135–159.

14 Pohontsch, N.J., Stark, A., Ehrhardt, M. et al. (2018) Influences on students' empathy in medical education: an exploratory interview study with medical students in their third and last year. *BMC Medical Education*, **18**, 231.

15 Uzogara, E.E., Lee, H., Abdou, C.M. and Jackson, J.S. (2014) A comparison of skin tone discrimination among African American men: 1995 and 2003. *Psychology of Men and Masculinities*, **15** (2), 201–212.

16 Medical Student Perspective: Medical School Survival: Replace Cut Throat Competition with Mutual Inspiration and Support. www.acponline.org/membership/medical-students/acp-impact/archive/june-2014/

medical-student-perspective-medical-school-survival-replace-cut-throat-competition-with-mutual (accessed 17th October 2022)

17 Orom, H., Semalulu, T. and Underwood, W. (2013) The social and learning environments experienced by underrepresented minority medical students. *Academic Medicine,* **88** (11), 1765–1777.

18 Jefferson, L., Bloor, K. and Maynard, A. (2015) Women in medicine: historical perspectives and recent trends. *British Medical Bulletin,* **114** (1), 5–15.

19 Togioka, B.M., Duvivier, D. and Young, E. (2022) Diversity and discrimination in healthcare. In: *StatPearls.* Treasure Island, FL: StatPearls Publishing. www.ncbi.nlm.nih.gov/books/NBK568721

20 Nazar, M., Kendall, K., Day, L. and Nazar, H. (2015) Decolonising medical curricula through diversity education: lessons from students. *Medical Teacher,* **37** (4), 385–393.

CHAPTER 6

Women in Healthcare

Olivia O'Connell[1] and Anna Frain[2]

[1] GP Teaching Fellow, University of Nottingham, Nottingham, UK; General Practitioner, Derby, UK;
[2] Programme Director Derby Speciality Training Scheme for General Practice, Derby, UK; General Practitioner, Derby, UK; GP Teaching Fellow, University of Nottingham, Nottingham, UK.

OVERVIEW

- While women represent over 70% of the global healthcare workforce, less than 25% are senior healthcare leaders.
- Historically, female clinicians and academics have been less prominent as researchers.
- Often, female patients have been excluded from research.
- A gender pay gap adversely affects female clinicians' careers.
- In some diseases, such as heart disease, health outcomes for women are worse than for men.
- Female patients' symptoms may be taken less seriously due to bias among clinicians.

Introduction

Women's health is affected by discrimination in research, knowledge of disease in women and inequality in treatment. Female clinicians' careers are affected adversely by a lack of equality in training and progression. Sexism and sexual harassment blight patients and clinicians. This chapter explores the evidence for historical and present-day issues and considers future developments.

Historical perspective

There is a perceived association of the female with instability, irrationality and excessive emotion. These attitudes are prevalent in healthcare.

> 'The feminization of madness is crazy.'
>
> (Gary Nunn [1])

Terminology sets the tone.

- The word 'hysteria' comes from *hystericus*, meaning 'of the womb'.
- Hysterectomy is the removal of the womb.
- 'Looney' is derived from lunacy, a monthly insanity akin to periods.

Delay in diagnosis due to assumptions of mental health issues, failure to listen and lack of knowledge of illness in women causes unnecessary morbidity and mortality [2,3]. Female pioneers faced barriers

entering the profession during training and once qualified. Initially, clinical specialties were open only to men. Reacting to female students being barred from clinics, Ann Preston, first woman dean of a US medical school, responded:

> 'Wherever it is proper to introduce women as patients, there also is it but just … for women to appear as physicians and students.'
>
> (Ann Preston 1813–1872 [4])

Issues concerning career choice, progression, bias and sexual harassment remain. Historically, clinical research has been based on data from trials involving male patients' conditions. Implications include a lack of appreciation of different disease patterns (e.g. cardiology), the metabolism of drugs and the efficacy of treatments in women [2].

Barriers to women in healthcare

Barriers exist to women's advancement in healthcare globally. These include the triple burdens of domestic, clinical and leadership roles. Gender bias, the gender pay gap, lack of flexible working arrangements, lack of mentoring and confidence, work/life balance, culture and stereotypes all affect advancement in leadership for women (Table 6.1) [5].

Career choice

While men have been at the forefront of clinical medicine, research and education, female pioneers in healthcare had to fight for recognition of their roles and contributions. Historically, many specialties and leadership roles were limited to men and not accessible to women (Table 6.2).

In the UK, 55% of medical students are female, with 36.6% of consultant-level doctors being women [6]. Improvements have required innovative solutions and required women leaders to address historical issues (Box 6.1). Reasons are multifactorial but include gender stereotypes and implicit and explicit gender bias [7].

Box 6.1 **Women in healthcare leadership.**

Dr Mumtaz Patel, Global Vice-president of the Royal College of Physicians (RCP), has helped develop the Global Women's Leaders

---

ABC of Equality, Diversity and Inclusion in Healthcare, First Edition. Edited by Shehla Imtiaz-Umer and John Frain.
© 2023 John Wiley & Sons Ltd. Published 2023 by John Wiley & Sons Ltd.

Programme. It aims to address the imbalance in leadership opportunities for women to motivate and inspire them to take on leadership roles within their healthcare organisations by providing mentorship and connection for women worldwide. By promoting system and organisational change, female talent can be preserved.

Historically, women at the top of organisations have been known to change the culture and improve organisational performance and patient care. This underlines the importance of having programmes specifically empowering the female healthcare workforce.

Source: Royal College of Physicians. Women in Health Care Leadership. www.rcp.org.uk

Table 6.1 Barriers to women in leadership positions across healthcare, academia and business [5].

Leadership barrier	Prevalence (%)		
	Healthcare	Academia	Business
Gender gap	12	12	10
Lack of career opportunities	12	10	7
Impact of stereotyping	10	8	12
Work/life balance	9	10	10
Lack of mentoring	10	11	6
Lack of flexible working environment	7	10	6
Gender bias	5	7	8
Lack of confidence	7	5	3
Leadership skills	5	5	3
Workplace culture	2	3	6
Gender pay gap	1	4	4
Race discrimination	1	2	5
Sexual harassment	1	0	0

Researchers calculated the frequency of each barrier occurring in the literature systematically reviewed for each profession. A 'barriers thematic map' estimated the prevalence of each barrier across the professions. Source: Adapted from Kalaitzi, S., Czabanowska, K., Fowler-Davis, S. and Brand, H. (2017) Women leadership barriers in healthcare, academia and business. Equality, Diversity and Inclusion, **36**(5), 457–474.

Table 6.2 Historical timeline for women in medicine.

Date	Notable female achievement
2050 BCE	Ubartum, female physician in Mesopotamia
Fourth century BCE	Agnodice, first female physician of ancient Athens
c. 200–400 CE	Metrodona, Greek physician. 'On the diseases and cures of women' was first medical text attributed to a woman
1151–58	Hildegard of Bingen, Germany's first female physician
1273–1410	24 women surgeons in Naples
1387–1497	15 women practitioners in Germany; most were Jewish
1849	Elizabeth Blackwell, born in England – first woman doctor in the United States. Graduated from New York in 1849. Co-founded the New York Infirmary for Women and Children

Table 6.2 (Continued)

Date	Notable female achievement
2050 BCE	Ubartum, female physician in Mesopotamia
1864	Rebecca Lee Crumpler – first African-American female physician in the USA
1865	Elizabeth Garrett Anderson, physician and surgeon – first female doctor in the UK who co-founded the London School of Medicine for Women
1870	Frances Hoggan – first female doctor in Wales
1878	Sophie Jex-Blake – first woman to practise medicine in Scotland. Co-founded both the London School of Medicine for Women and the Edinburgh School of Medicine in 1874
1899	China's Hu King Eng graduated in Ohio and returned to work in Fuzhou
1952	Annis Gillie, founder member of the RCGP, UK and College Chair 1959–1962. First female vice-chair of the British Medical Association (BMA)
1959	Sheila Sherlock – first female professor of medicine in the UK
1961	Dame Cicely Saunders – founder of the Hospice Movement
1985	Margaret Allen – first woman heart transplant surgeon in the US
1989	Margaret Turner Warwick – first female President of the Royal College of Physicians (RCP). 'I had no wish to be any kind of feminist or pioneer or curiosity. That would have got in the way; gender has no place in Medicine.' The RCP was founded in 1518, and of a total of 120 presidents, three have been women.
2008	First Tuvaluan female doctors
2010	Dame Sally Davies – first female Chief Medical Officer in the UK
2019	Clare Marx – first woman chair of the General Medical Council (GMC)
2021	Farah Jameel elected first female chair of the BMA GP Committee (GPC) in its 100-year history

UK female medical students today report experiencing adverse comments due to their gender and proposed specialty choice (Box 6.2). A BMA survey demonstrates this as an ongoing issue affecting career choice (Table 6.3) [8]. Gender inequality affects significantly more women than men.

Box 6.2 **'Why are you training to be a doctor?'**

'I have been asked whether and why I am sacrificing a personal life/chance for a family by choosing medicine as a career. I've been told (separately by a patient and a consultant) that I will have no problem finding a nice male doctor to settle down with. I have been given lots of advice on "how to have it all" and how to choose a career/training path that allows me to also have a family of my own.

I was part of a conversation where a female surgeon informed my colleague and I that, as women, if we were sensitive, we would not

survive in medicine. We were informed that we would have to be tough to succeed as a female hospital doctor.'
Zoe Blyde, Graduate Entry Medical Student.

Seniority and the gender pay gap

The UK Royal College of Nursing (RCN) reported that the gender pay gap is related to the more significant proportion of men in senior roles, not the rates of pay for men and women doing similar work (see Further resources). Women are likelier to be less than full time (LTFT), with a reduction in overall lifetime earnings and pension. Hospital doctors have the most significant gap at 18.9%, with GPs at 15.3% and clinical academics at 11.9%. This is adjusted for contracted hours. The gender pay gap increases with age [9].

In the UK, 73% of Clinical Excellence Awards (CEA) went to men in 2019. These involve pensionable pay increases. The percentage of male and female success rates for CEA applications is similar, and scoring mechanisms are unbiased towards either gender. However, female consultants are underrepresented, especially for higher-level awards [10].

'Given the ladder structure of the current award process, holders of the higher CEA, e.g. gold and platinum, will be inevitably older – and because of the composition of the workforce, more likely to be white and male compared to those holding bronze or local awards.' [11]

The current system is being reformed, aiming to broaden access and make application to the scheme fairer and more inclusive.

Academia

The COVID-19 pandemic has created additional challenges and a reduction in academic output for female academics [12]. Before this,

whilst a gender gap in research roles existed, the proportion of female authors increased from 32% to 41% from 2000 to 2015 but was still well below 50% [13].

Training

For both sexes, training in healthcare is challenging while caring for children or relatives, during ill health or under personal stress. Moving for training placements, juggling clinical work and studying for exams can strain personal and family lives. Some LTFT trainees have encountered hostility, difficulty meeting training needs, pay and rota problems, and a lack of support in returning to work after a period of absence.

It is suggested that training in medicine involves accepting a system biased against women, with notable absences of women in specific fields, for example some fields of psychiatry. Twenty-eight percent of male respondents to the BMA's 'Sexism in medicine' report felt they had had more opportunities during training because of their gender compared to only 1% of women (Table 6.3) [8]. Seventy per cent of female respondents felt their clinical ability had been doubted or undervalued because of their gender, compared to 12% of men. Seventy-four percent of all respondents thought sexism was a barrier to career progression.

Awareness of gender inequality in healthcare is improving. Women in leadership roles report that male colleagues supported them in their careers and flexible training, providing mentorship and role models. The value of workplace mentors of either gender and support networks in juggling work and family life is acknowledged. They encourage reapplication after an unsuccessful job and CEA award application, stepping outside one's comfort zone, not fearing failure, understanding imposter syndrome and being brave as a female leader (see Further resources, NUH 2022). Women's mentorship can provide networking, encouragement, opportunities and empowerment (Box 6.3, Box 6.4) [14].

Table 6.3 Summary of findings of the Sexism in Medicine report [8].

- 91% of women respondents had experienced sexism at work within the past two years.

- 84% of all respondents said there was an issue of sexism in the medical profession.

- 28% of men respondents said that they have/had more opportunities during training because of their gender, in comparison to 1% of women respondents.

- 74% of all respondents think that sexism acts as a barrier to career progression.

- 42% of all respondents who witnessed or experienced an issue relating to sexism in the past two years chose not to raise it with anyone.

- 61% of women felt they were discouraged to work in a particular specialty because of their gender, with 39% going on to not work in that specialty.

- 70% of women respondents felt that their clinical ability had been doubted or undervalued because of their gender, in comparison to 12% of men.

- 31% of women respondents experienced unwanted physical conduct in the workplace as did 23% of men respondents.

- 56% of women respondents had received unwanted verbal conduct relating to their gender, as did 28% of men respondents.

Box 6.3 **'I wish I'd known before …'**

'I think the things I have learnt/wish I had done better/known are:
- Imposter syndrome is "normal". I've been a consultant surgeon for 15 years and still feel like the new girl who will be found out!
- As a mother and surgeon, you will always feel guilty that you are not giving 100% to either half of your life, but that's OK and normal.
- You can't please everyone, and saying no is allowed.
- Good-quality childcare is essential, as is a backup plan for when you can't do the pickup on time…. Good friends and family can help, but only if you ask!'
Miss Alison Payne, Consultant Colorectal Surgeon.

Box 6.4 **'Find a mentor – or two.'**

'As I moved through my career, I've seen lots of great practice, but also some not great practice (clinically but also in how to behave/ teamwork/supervising). Good role models are so important. Educational supervisors (ES) try to fit this into junior doctors' practice, but you may "click" with people who aren't your ES. They might be your peer but are usually higher up the career ladder, and I've loved

being a mentor and made lifelong friendships with those who were *my* mentors. I think that this is especially important for us ladies. For years the men have had their own "old boys' clubs", and us supporting one other is such a great thing to be part of.'
    Dr Sarah Russ, Consultant Anaesthetist.

Challenges for female healthcare workers

Women in healthcare may experience challenges relating to stages of their reproductive life.

Periods

There is increasing awareness of difficulties coping with periods in clinical settings, particularly with long shifts, operations or prolonged time in PPE. Suggestions include introducing universally dark colour scrubs, provision of period products in clinical areas, and recommendations for free menstrual products by theatre and intensive care departments [15].

Fertility and pregnancy

Trying to conceive may also be difficult, with infertility among doctors higher than in the general population. Healthcare workers may simultaneously take exams, move for placements, decide their career pathway or apply for jobs. Undergoing assisted conception raises practical issues around shift work and rotas, including the timing of cycles, implantation and emotional stress. One recommendation is that a departmental lead for health in fertility and pregnancy can support and advocate for rota or working pattern modification [15].

Healthcare workers who have experienced pregnancy loss and assisted conception may also be working in roles requiring them to support patients in the same position. Colleagues or supervisors may not always realise the emotional difficulty of this. Healthcare workers may have concerns regarding risks to mother and baby posed by clinical environments.

The NHS trade unions' information, and guidance on COVID-19, acknowledge that risks to pregnant women in the health service include manual handling, radiation, infectious diseases, toxic chemicals, shift work and mental and physical fatigue (see Further resources). Adoption leave may cause stress and anxiety in female and male healthcare workers, with the process involving taking leave at short notice.

Breastfeeding

Many NHS staff feel unable to breastfeed, despite recommendations that employers provide basic provisions for women to express milk at work. NHS employees express milk in toilets, stairwells and broom cupboards; many women stop breastfeeding due to workplace difficulties. They face humiliating comments from colleagues, lack of breaks to express milk, leaking of milk and lack of storage for expressing equipment [16]. This is despite 77% of the NHS' 1.7 million strong workforce being women. In the UK, breastfeeding rates are among the lowest in the world.

Menopause

In her 'Wellness Compendium', Dr Susie Hewitt explains that menopause occurs when female clinicians are at the peak of their careers (see Further resources). Flushes, sleep deprivation and emotional changes

can have adverse effects. Materials from the British Menopause Society and the Royal College of Obstetricians and Gynaecologists can help workplaces meet the needs of their workforce (see Further resources).

The Chartered Society of Physiotherapy (CSP) website acknowledges that physiotherapy is a female-dominated profession and that managers should conduct risk assessments concerning menopause and perimenopause. Their website includes an Equality and Diversity Toolkit (see Further resources).

Sexism and harassment

The BMA has recently been subject to publicity regarding the GP Committee chairperson, who faced sexist comments and poor conduct which affected her health and wellbeing. Two unrelated independent reviews also highlighted a culture of sexism within the BMA (Box 6.5).

Box 6.5 **Sexism at the BMA.**

In 2021, Farah Jameel was elected the first female chair of the BMA GP committee in its 100-year history. She experienced sexism within the first few months of the job. The 'conduct and culture' of the BMA resulted in her needing to take sick leave.

Previous similar allegations of sexism occurred in 2019. A report by Daphne Romney QC found there was an 'old boys' network. A further report in 2022 by Ijeoma Omambala (commissioned prior to Dr Jameel's experience) reported that 'rude, bullying and disrespectful' behaviour was potentially contributing to the marginalisation of women, ethnic minorities and other minority voices in national and local GP committees.

Sources: Romney, D. (2019) Independent Report into Sexism at the BMA. www.bma.org.uk/media/1244/bma-daphne-romney-qc-report-oct-19.pdf. Omambala, I. (2022) Independent review of the current representative structure of general practitioners in the UK. www.gpdf.org.uk/wp-content/uploads/2022/05/GPDF-IOQC-Report-Final-070522.pdf

---

Dr Chelcie Jewitt experienced sexism and saw her colleagues endure much worse levels of misogyny, assault and discrimination. She started with a small survey on social media and presented it to colleagues. With the support of the BMA, this developed into the 2021 Sexism in Medicine report [8]. Her experiences and those of many other clinicians are reflected also in the experiences of female medical students (Box 6.6, Box 6.7, Box 6.8, Box 6.9).

Box 6.6 **It is not how it's intended; it is how it is received by the victim.**

During her first clinical attachment, Harriet complained about a senior doctor. He had made inappropriate comments directly to her when only two nurses were in the room. After looking her up and down, he had bemoaned that medical students had to wear scrubs and not the type of uniforms that nurses wore in the past. He said those were better as they were more revealing. Despite being told the complaint would be taken seriously, it was dropped. The investigators felt the comment had not been malicious. Harriet felt isolated and upset. She felt she could not take her concerns any further; otherwise, she would be labelled a troublemaker. She was shocked that this had happened in the NHS today.

Box 6.7 **Mistaken identity.**

James, an ST1* doctor, visited a ward unfamiliar to him to see a patient who had been handed over to him. Once James had seen the patient, he wished to speak to the consultant on ward round that day to update them. He went toward the nurses' station and identified a male clinician dressed in scrubs, whom he assumed was the consultant with his juniors huddled around him. James introduced himself to the clinician and began giving him an update regarding his patient. The man seemed to look confused when James spoke to him. Shortly after, one of the female doctors wearing scrubs stood up from behind the computer, stating that she was, in fact, the consultant. She said James should not have assumed that her registrar was the consultant because he was a male.

*A doctor in the first year of specialty training (ST).

Box 6.8 **Ingrained gender roles.**

Priya, a third-year medical student, observed a stent insertion in the catheter lab. Sophie, a student paramedic, was also observing the procedure. They chatted about what year they were in at university, and Priya asked how much longer Sophie had left until she qualified. Sophie asked Priya the same question and was confused when she said she still had another 2.5 years to go. 'I thought nurses only studied for three years before they qualified,' she said. Priya, who had already been mistaken for a nurse multiple times over her short placement, sighed and said, 'No, I'm training to be a doctor. Women can be doctors too, you know'.

Box 6.9 **Lost hope for the future of women in healthcare?**

During a lunch break, fourth-year medical students Rehan and Amina were discussing the differences in how they have been treated by other medical professionals and patients while on their clinical placement thus far. Amina was expressing her frustration about being a woman in healthcare. Rehan explained that he wished women were given equal opportunities to men but that the reality is that female doctors are unlikely to be even considered equal to men for another 30+ years. If he were given an opportunity on the premise of being male despite his female colleague being better for the role, he would take it to further his career without a second thought.

These stories are consistent with experiences for other healthcare workers. The International Confederation of Midwives reported that 10% of female midwives had experienced sexual harassment at work. These women reported that superiors did not adequately support them, and no actions were taken against the offender.

The explicit devaluing of female healthcare assistants (HCAs) in financial terms was reported in 'Surviving in Scrubs', an online space founded by Dr Chelcie Jewitt that allows women to anonymously share their experiences of sexual assault, harassment and discrimination in healthcare workplaces. It aims to raise awareness and campaign to end this culture.

Tackling these issues is essential and urgent. Training in allyship and being an active bystander can empower young clinicians (see Chapter 12). However, without the training of established professionals, change will not happen

Women's health

'Medicine must hear unwell women when they speak – not as females but as human beings. Medicine must listen to and believe our testimonies about our own bodies, and ultimately turn its energies, time, and money towards finally solving our medical mysteries. The answers reside in our bodies, and in the histories our bodies have always been writing.'

(Elinor Cleghorn [3])

Research

Until the late 1990s, much research developing our understanding and treatment of disease, use of drugs and interventions had taken place on male patients [3]. Female patients were studied for diseases of the breast and reproductive organs. Drugs and interventions studied in men produce different results in women in some diseases, leading to poorer outcomes. Heart disease, a significant public health issue in the late twentieth century, is a good example.

Similar research biases have occurred about age and ethnicity (see Chapters 2 and 4). In the 1990s, research funding by the National Institutes of Health in the USA became dependent on more inclusive research design and reporting of outcomes (Box. 6.10).

Box 6.10 **The National Institutes of Health (NIH) Revitalization Act, 1993.**

The NIH has stewardship for medical research in the United States. Its mission is to seek, extend and apply knowledge of living systems to enhance health, lengthen life and reduce illness and disability. Historically, however, women and minority groups were excluded from research.

The Act required the NIH to establish legally binding guidance for NIH-funded researchers to include women, including those of childbearing age, and ethnic/racial minorities into studies and clinical trials. The Act forbids exclusion of these groups on grounds of cost particularly in relation to clinical research and clinical trials.

Women and heart disease

Hypertension is a risk factor for heart disease in women, yet only 25% of women with hypertension are treated adequately [2]. Hypertension is often symptomatic in women and listening to and treating them effectively is essential as women are often ignored. Gathering information about simple factors such as family history, history of migraines at a young age and pre-eclampsia can lead to earlier diagnosis and better treatment. The concerns of women with heart disease are often ignored. The understanding of different patterns of atherosclerosis and the ageing of the heart muscle between women and men has grown gradually. Afro-Caribbean women have high blood pressure at a younger age, increased prevalence of enlarged heart muscle and more hypertension in pregnancy [2].

'Typical' presentations of heart disease taught to students and clinicians are based on research in male patients (usually white Caucasian males weighing 70 kg), leading to the 'atypical' presentations of female patients not being recognised, misinterpreted and resulting in worse outcomes. There has been a developing understanding of the bias in teaching students for many years, yet female patients still experience poor care and results. Table 6.4 shows the historical timeline of how the understanding of female heart disease has developed.

Box 6.11 summarises study conclusions regarding female patients presenting with typical and atypical chest pain. Perhaps the terms 'typical' and 'atypical' should be retired as they help to continue the stereotype.

Box 6.11 Does the chest pain of acute coronary syndrome (ACS) present differently in women compared to men?

Cardiac chest pain, we are taught, typically presents as a crushing, heavy, dull sensation in the middle of the chest which then radiates to the left arm. If the pain is not like this then it may be attributed to a non-cardiac cause such as muscular or anxiety related. This may delay accurate diagnosis and treatment.

'I encountered a female patient in her 50s presenting with a possible acute coronary syndrome (ACS). We had recently been discussing in clinical skills possible differences in the presentation of an acute coronary syndrome in women and men and how this can affect outcomes for women. I decided to examine the evidence for this. I undertook a systematic search of the literature using the 6S evidence pyramid we had been taught. I identified 16 relevant studies using the SORT criteria.* I was able to draw the following conclusions.

- Women are more likely to present with ACS atypically compared to men.
- Men are more likely to present with chest pain than women.
- Chest pain is the most common symptom presentation for both sexes.
- Younger women are more likely than older women to present with typical symptoms.
- No difference exists between sexes for the prevalence of chest pain and/or other typical symptoms of ACS.
- Women reported more associated (non-chest pain) ACS symptoms than men.'

*Ebell, M.H., Siwek, J., Weiss, B.D. et al. (2004) Strength of recommendation taxonomy (SORT): a patient-centered approach to grading evidence in the medical literature. *American Family Physician*, **69**(3), 548–556.

This is an excerpt from a patient-based piece of coursework undertaken by Graduate Entry Medicine students at the University of Nottingham, UK.

Lucille Middleton, Graduate Entry Medical student

Source: Adapted from Box 2.1, *ABC of Clinical Reasoning*, 2nd edn, 2023.

Table 6.4 Historical developments in the understanding of heart disease in women.

1772	William Heberden Angina defined as chest pains in men older than 50 years Women typically died in childbirth or before symptoms developed
1960s	Portland, Oregon. Teaching women how to support their husbands with their heart attack [2]
1973	Women demanded too much from their husbands leading to heart disease (Skelton, BMJ)
1973	Coronary Drug Project: Oestrogen trial Trial treating more than 8000 men with oestrogen or placebo (based on the assumption that it protected women against heart disease) was stopped due to higher mortality in men on higher doses of oestrogen. This led to an understanding that the role of oestrogen was much more complex.
1991	Breakthrough research articles on cardiovascular disease in women in the *New England Journal of Medicine* (Legato MJ et al., Ayanian JZ, Steingart RM) Marianne Legato wished to end the misperception of women with symptoms of heart disease as hysterical
1990–2000s	Women's Ischaemic Syndrome Evaluation (WISE) studies specifically researched the mechanisms of heart disease in women
2009	Professor Londa Scheibinger launched 'Gendered innovations'. She aimed to integrate the theme 'sex and gender' into all science and technology sectors.
2013	European Commission published guidelines for the implementation of sex and gender aspects in all research commissioned by the European Union
2015	In Holland, the Gender and Health Alliance set up a Knowledge Agenda. They highlighted gaps in appropriate effective care for women, resulting in funding and research. Cardiovascular health was a priority.
2019	'A Woman's Heart' by Angela Maas was published in Holland

The gender of the clinician can affect treatment. This includes female physicians adhering more closely to guidelines than men, fewer complications and a lower risk of dying post heart attack if treated by a female.

Women, delayed diagnoses and poor treatment

Elinor Cleghorn outlines the struggles she experienced over seven years, waiting to receive a diagnosis for her ill health [3]. Often, this results from a failure to listen to women's symptoms. Menopause is blamed for many symptoms suffered by women. In her 2020 report on the impact of medical devices on women's health, 'First, do no Harm', Baroness Julia Cumberlege commented:

'Anything and everything women suffer (tends to be…) perceived as a natural precursor to, part of or a post-symptomatic phase of the menopause.' [17]

There are numerous examples of delayed diagnoses.

- Endometriosis affects 10% of reproductive age women globally.
- Average time to diagnosis from onset of symptoms to diagnosis is eight years (UK) with Black and minority ethnic communities facing additional barriers [18].
- Chronic fatigue syndrome/ME affects more women than men (4:1).
- Fibromyalgia male:female ratio is 1:9. Mean time to diagnosis is 6.42 years [19].
- Gynaecology waiting lists have faced the biggest increase of all medical specialties in England, with one in 20 facing a year-long wait for treatment (see Further resources).

Women and mental health

Around one in five women in the UK have a mental health (MH) problem; gender-specific risk factors include the likelihood of women being carers, experiencing physical or sexual abuse or living in poverty. However, protective factors for women's mental health include better support networks than men, ease of confiding in friends and being more likely to seek help for a MH problem. This help seeking is thought to protect women from suicide; 1 in 4 of those who complete suicide are women.

The risk of dangerous arrhythmias when taking a combination of antibiotics and psychiatry medications is more significant in women than in men.

The COVID-19 pandemic has amplified MH difficulties in healthcare workers with post-traumatic stress disorder (PTSD), anxiety and burnout. Suicide rates amongst female doctors are twice those of the general female population, with patient complaints contributing significantly. Barriers to doctors of both genders seeking help for MH include stigma, professional implications, taking on a 'patient' role and time off work.

A systematic review showed that, in general, female GPs were more likely to have longer consultation lengths, were less likely to prescribe, more likely to write longer records and less likely to refer [20]. These factors may contribute to stress/burnout in females, which is currently prevalent throughout the UK GP workforce.

Gender bias and racism

Gender bias and structural racism make toxic companions (see Chapters 2 and 4). In the US, 22% of ethnic minority women experience discrimination when visiting a doctor or clinic. In the UK, Black women are five times more likely to die in childbirth than Caucasians [21]. Hoffman reported how racist myths about pain perception in Black people led to disparities in the treatment of ethnic minority women's pain, including being given less analgesia and potentially fatal delays in diagnoses such as pre-eclampsia, which persist today [22].

Conclusion

Angela Maas reports significant developments in the understanding and treatment of heart disease in women over the last 25 years [2]. This is encouraging but there remain many areas of women's health where lack of knowledge, the inability of clinicians to listen to female patients and bias, both implicit and explicit, still result in increased morbidity and mortality. The UK government's Women's Health Strategy (see Further resources) is a positive development although its impact is still unknown (Table 6.5).

Table 6.5 Summary of women's health strategy for England, 2021.

Priority areas	Strategy
Menstrual health and gynaecological conditions	Improve awareness and care of these conditions
Fertility, pregnancy, pregnancy loss and post-natal support	Empower women to make choices about their reproduction
The menopause	A holistic approach to improving care and support
Healthy ageing and long-term conditions	Extending healthy life expectancy by five years by 2035, reduce the gap between rich and poor
Mental health	Examine factors which impact women's mental health
The health impacts of violence against women and girls	Build evidence and improve support and safety
84% of respondents described instances in which they had not been listened to by healthcare professionals	Better understand why doctors don't listen to women
Services for specialties or conditions which only or primarily affect women, for example, reproductive health services are perceived to be of a lower priority compared to other services	Joint commissioning, innovative models of care, reduction of disparities
Healthcare professionals need to receive better education and training on women's health conditions	Improved teaching in schools, digital information and support for GPs to implement guidelines
Health conditions and disabilities can affect women's experience in the workplace and can increase women's stress levels, impacting their mental health and productivity	Flexible working, improved workplace support, workplace menopause policy
Lack of research into women's health and subsequent lack of data	Increase research into women's health, looking specifically at sex differences in conditions. Improve diversity of research participants

Source: Women's Health Strategy. www.gov.uk/government/publications/womens-health-strategy-for-england

Today's female students and healthcare workers still experience bias, harassment and prejudice. Careers and lives are still adversely affected, and much work must be done.

Acknowledgement

Thank you to the following contributors: Dr Sarah Russ, Miss Alison Payne, Consultants, and Graduate Entry Medical students Lucille Middleton and Zoe Blyde.

Further reading/resources

Baumhäkel, M., Müller, U., Böhm, M. (2009) Influence of gender of physicians and patients on guideline-recommended treatment of chronic heart failure in a cross-sectional study. *European Journal of Heart Failure*, **11** (3), 299–303.

Chartered Society of Physiotherapists Equality and Diversity Toolkit. www.csp.org.uk/publications/equality-diversity-toolkit-practical-guide-csp-stewards-managers-members (accessed 06 September 2022)

Hewitt, S. and Kennedy, U. (2019). *EM-POWER: A Wellness Compendium for EM*. London: Royal College of Emergency Medicine. https://rcem.ac.uk/wp-content/uploads/2021/10/Wellness_Compendium_June2019.pdf (accessed 1 October 2022)

NUH Women in Medicine – an International Women's Day inspired talk. www.youtube.com/watch?v=ZVCAJNG2lHs&ab_channel=NUHonYoutube (accessed 12 October 2022)

Priori, S.G., Schwartz, P.J., Napolitano, C. et al.(2003) Risk stratification in the long-QT syndrome. *New England Journal of Medicine*, **348** (19), 1866–1874.

Regan, L. (2021) Better for women. Improving the health and wellbeing of girls and women. Towards a women's health strategy for the UK. *European Journal of Public Health*, **31** (Supplement_3). (accessed 2 October 2022)

Royal College of Psychiatrists: 25 Women Project www.rcpsych.ac.uk/members/special-interest-groups/women-and-mental-health/25-women-project (accessed 2 October 2022)

Royal College of Obstetricians and Gynaecologists (2022) Left for too long: understanding the scale and impact of gynaecology waiting lists. www.rcog.org.uk/about-us/campaigning-and-opinions/left-for-too-long-understanding-the-scale-and-impact-of-gynaecology-waiting-lists (accessed 2 October 2022)

Surviving in Scrubs https://survivinginscrubsorg.wordpress.com (accessed 2 October 2022)

Tsugawa, Y., Jena, A.B., Figueroa, J.F., Orav, E.J., Blumenthal, D.M. and Jha, A.K. (2017) Comparison of hospital mortality and readmission rates for medicare patients treated by male vs female physicians. *JAMA Internal Medicine*, **177** (2), 206–213.

Wilson, A. and Childs, S. (2002) The relationship between consultation length, process, and outcomes in general practice: a systematic review. *British Journal of General Practice*, **52** (485), 1012–1020. PMID: 12528590; PMCID: PMC1314474.

Women's Health Strategy www.gov.uk/government/publications/womens-health-strategy-for-england (accessed 2 October 2022)

References

1 Nunn, G. (20212) The feminisation of madness is crazy. The Guardian, London. www.theguardian.com/media/mind-your-language/2012/mar/08/mind-your-language-feminisation-madness (accessed 01 October 2022)

2 Maas, A. (2020) *A Woman's Heart*. London: Aster.

3 Cleghorn, E. (2021) *Unwell Women*. London: Weidenfeld and Nicolson.

4 Weiner, S. (2020) Celebrating 10 Women Medical Pioneers. www.aamc.org/news-insights/celebrating-10-women-medical-pioneers (accessed 01 October 2022)

5 Kalaitzi, S., Czabanowska, K., Fowler-Davis, S. and Brand, H. (2017) Women leadership barriers in healthcare, academia and business. *Equality Diversity and Inclusion*, **36** (5), 457–474.

6 General Medical Council (2019) The state of medical education and practice in the UK. London: General Medical Council.

7 Salles, A., Awad, M., Goldin, L. et al. (2019) Estimating implicit and explicit gender bias among health care professionals and surgeons. *JAMA Network Open*, **2** (7), e196545.

8 British Medical Association (2021) *Sexism in Medicine*. London: BMA.

9 Department of Health and Social Care (2020) *Mend the Gap: The Independent Review into Gender Pay Gaps in Medicine in England*. London: Department of Health and Social Care.

10 Advisory Committee on Clinical Excellence Awards (2020) www.gov.uk/government/organisations/advisory-committee-on-clinical-excellence-awards (accessed 01 October 2022)

11 BMA (2021) *Consultation on the reform of the national clinical excellence awards scheme. BMA response*. www.bma.org.uk/media/5527/bma-response-to-accea-consultation-on-nceas.pdf (accessed 01 October 2022)

12 Gabster, B.P., van Daalen, K., Dhatt, R. and Barry, M. (2020) Challenges for the female academic during the COVID-19 pandemic. *Lancet*, **395** (10242), 1968–1970.

13 Gayet-Ageron, A., Poncet, A. and Perneger, T. (2019) Comparison of the contributions of female and male authors to medical research in 2000 and 2015: a cross-sectional study. *BMJ Open*, **9** (2), e024436.

14 Loethen, J. and Ananthamurugan, M. (2021) Women in medicine: the quest for mentorship. *Missouri Medicine*, **118** (3), 182–184.

15 Critchley, J., Schwarz, M. and Baruah, R. (2021) The female medical workforce. *Anaesthesia*, **76**: 14–23.

16 Hearfield, H., Collier, J. and Paize, F. (2022) Breast feeding experiences of NHS staff returning to work from maternity leave: a national study. *BJPsych Open*, **8** (S1), S53–4.

17 Cumberlege, J. (2020) First do no harm: the report of the independent medicines and medical devices safety review. www.immdsreview.org.uk/Report.html (accessed 02 October 2022)

18 (2020) Endometriosis in the UK: time for change an APPG on endometriosis inquiry report. www.endometriosisuk.org/sites/default/files/files/Endometriosis%20APPG%20Report%20Oct%202020.pdf (accessed 02 October 2022)

19 Bartels, E.M., Dreyer, L., Jacobsen, S. et al. (2009) Fibromyalgi, diagnostik og praevalens. Kan kønsforskellen forklares? [Fibromyalgia, diagnosis, and prevalence. Are gender differences explainable?]. *Ugeskr Laeger*, **171** (49), 3588–3592.

20 Wilson, A. and Childs, S. (2002) The relationship between consultation length, process, and outcomes in general practice: a systematic review. *British Journal of General Practice*, **52** (485), 1012–1020.

21 MBRRACE (2019) MBRRACE-UK perinatal mortality surveillance report. www.npeu.ox.ac.uk/assets/downloads/mbrrace-uk/reports/perinatal-surveillance-report-2019/MBRRACE-UK_Perinatal_Surveillance_Report_2019_-_Final_v2.pdf.

22 Hoffman, K.M., Trawalter, S., Axt, J.R. and Oliver, M.N. (2016) Racial bias in pain assessment and treatment recommendations, and false beliefs about biological differences between blacks and whites. *Proceedings of the National Academy of Sciences USA*, **113** (16), 4296–4301.

CHAPTER 7

Sexual Orientation and Gender Identity

Duncan McGregor

Core Trainee Doctor, North West School of Anaesthetics, Manchester, UK
LGBTQ+ Health Activist, Ex-Chair for GLADD – Association of LGBTQ+ Doctors and Dentists, London, UK

OVERVIEW

- A patient's sexuality and gender identity are relevant to their care.
- Healthcare professionals should understand:
  - definitions of sex, gender and sexuality
  - common sexual orientations and gender identities
  - key trends of LGBTQ+ health inequalities
  - practising allyship with respect to LGBTQ+ issues in healthcare.
- Healthcare professionals can improve the inclusivity of health services for LGBTQ+ patients and staff.

Introduction and history

The LGBTQ+ rights movement is relatively recent compared to other civil rights movements. With male homosexual acts decriminalised in the UK only in 1967, it is within living memory that simply being homosexual, or bisexual, was a punishable criminal offence. Following Margaret Thatcher's speech stating that children 'are being taught that they have an inalienable right to be gay', the introduction of Section 28 in the UK in 1988 prohibited the 'promotion of homosexuality' by local authorities, effectively banning education on sexuality in schools until its repeal in 2003. Only in 2013, with the release of the *Diagnostic and Statistical Manual of Mental Disorders* version 5 (DSM-5), was it accepted that being transgender is not a mental pathology, the World Health Organization recognising this also in 2018.

As a result of Section 28, there is an entire generation of healthcare professionals who, throughout their entire education, received no formal teaching on LGBTQ+ matters. Lack of training about the LGBTQ+ experience is not unique to the UK. Healthcare professionals around the world have varying experience and understanding of issues relating to LGBTQ+ healthcare.

It is difficult to establish exactly how many LGBTQ+ people there are at any one time. Public Health England estimates that between 2.5% and 5.89% of the population identify as lesbian, gay or bisexual [1]. While there is no official statistic, the Gender Identity Research and Education Society estimate that approximately 1% of the population identifies as transgender or non-binary [2]. Given these

numbers and the close links between sexual orientation, gender identity and health inequalities, healthcare professionals need to have a working understanding of key aspects of LGBTQ+ topics.

Key terminology

Words used by healthcare professionals have long-lasting effects, with the choice of words remembered by patients for years or even their entire lives. The extensive LGBTQ+ terminology can be daunting when first approached. Table 7.1 shows a glossary of common terms. It is important not to feel overwhelmed by the terminology or afraid of using the wrong words. The aim is to enable the use of the appropriate words. We will consider some of these terms at greater length to provide a greater understanding.

Sex/gender

Sex and gender are terms often – incorrectly – used interchangeably. Sex relates to the biological characteristics of a person, historically categorised into 'male' and 'female' and based upon a person's chromosomes. Chromosomal compositions lead to differential hormonal profiles, which in turn cause external and internal primary and secondary sexual characteristics. These include the form and function of the internal and external genitalia, breast tissue development and body hair distribution patterns.

Gender is not related to underlying biological traits. It is related entirely to the sociocultural characteristics and identities of what it means to be a 'woman' or a 'man'. Historically, in Western culture, these characteristics and identities have linked the characteristics of being a man with that of the male sex, and likewise linked woman to that of being female. However, this is not a universal experience, and the roles and identities that society has expected of men and women differ between cultures at different times.

Sexual orientation

Sexual orientation or sexuality relates to the sexual and romantic attraction people feel towards others. The most common sexuality is heterosexual: sexual or romantic attraction to others of the opposite gender than oneself. Minority sexualities include (but are not limited

---

ABC of Equality, Diversity and Inclusion in Healthcare, First Edition. Edited by Shehla Imtiaz-Umer and John Frain.
© 2023 John Wiley & Sons Ltd. Published 2023 by John Wiley & Sons Ltd.

Table 7.1 Definitions and terminology related to LGBTQ+ identities and experience.

Term	Definition
Allosexual/ Alloromantic (Allo)	Allosexual people experience sexual attraction, and alloromantic people experience romantic attraction. Allo is to asexual and aromantic identities, as straight is to LGB+ spectrum identities. It is important to avoid using 'normal' as the opposite of asexual/aromantic identities, which is stigmatising.
Aromantic/Aro	Someone who experiences little to no *romantic* attraction. Aromantic people may or may not experience *sexual* attraction (see Asexual), and this sexual attraction may be in any orientation, e.g. homosexual, bisexual, etc.
Asexual/Ace	Someone who experiences little to no *sexual* attraction. Asexual people may or may not experience *romantic* attraction (see Aromantic), and this romantic attraction may be in any orientation, e.g. homoromantic, biromantic. etc. Asexual people may experience sexual pleasure but feel little to no sexual attraction to other people.
Ally	Someone who supports and advocates for equal civil rights and actively challenges discriminatory behaviour and institutions.
Bisexual/Bi	Someone who is sexually and/or romantically attracted to people of their own gender and those of a different gender. See also Pansexual.
Biphobia	The dislike of or prejudice specifically against bisexual people.
Butch/Masc	A descriptive term used for someone who expresses themselves in a typically masculine way. While it can and is often used as an affirmative label of identity expression, this term has been used in a derogatory manner for lesbians, so caution is advised in its use.
Cisgender/Cis	Someone whose gender identity matches the sex that they were assigned at birth.
Coming out	The act of first telling someone about one's sexual orientation/gender identity. This process may be repeated if meeting new people.
Deadnaming	A specific subclass of misgendering, deadnaming is to call someone by their birth name if they have changed it as part of their transition. This may be accidental or malicious and purposeful.
Femme/Fem	A descriptive term used for someone who expresses themselves in a typically feminine way.
Gay	Someone who is sexually and/or romantically attracted to people of their own gender. Gay is often used as an umbrella term for non-heterosexual sexual orientations; however, some homosexual women will identify as lesbian, not gay.
Gender	The identities and characteristics of women and men are socially constructed. The definitions and expectations of what it means to be of a given gender change between cultures and over time. Gender is a sociocultural expression of particular characteristics and roles associated with certain groups of people, often concerning their sex as assigned at birth.
Gender dysphoria	The feeling or experience of distress/discomfort provoked by the mismatch between sex assigned at birth and gender identity. Gender dysphoria is also the clinical diagnosis for this experience when distress impacts social, occupational or other important areas of functioning. Trans and non-binary gender identities are not in and of themselves a psychiatric condition.
Gender expression	The external and outwardly expression of one's gender, which may include use of specific pronouns, changes to name or expression through clothing, behaviour and body characteristics. This expression may or may not conform to societal expectations of gender.
Gender identity	One's innate, internal sense of one's own gender, which may or may not correspond to the sex assigned at birth.
Gender Recognition Certificate (GRC)	A document which changes an individual's legal gender, allowing their birth certificate to be reissued. This conveys the same legal rights and responsibilities conveyed on their new birth certificate. Not all trans people will apply for a GRC, and it is not required to change gender markers at work or to legally change gender on other documents such as a passport.
Heterosexual/straight	Someone who is sexually and/or romantically attracted to people of the opposite gender to their own.
Homosexual	Someone who is sexually and/or romantically attracted to people of their own gender. The terms 'gay' and 'lesbian' are now more generally used.
Homophobia	The dislike of or prejudice against homosexual people. Often used as an umbrella term to capture prejudice against all minority sexual orientations.
Intersex	Someone whose reproductive and sexual anatomy and/or physiology do not fit typical definitions of male or female sex due to a range of genetic and hormonal factors. Intersex people may or may not identify with the gender assigned to them at birth.
Intersectionality	The concept that people may have multiple overlapping identities which intersect different aspects of discrimination or privilege, and that civil rights movements and equality organisations must consider other marginalised identities. Of note is the higher burden of discrimination and prejudice experienced by multiply marginalised individuals.

Table 7.1 (Continued)

Term	Definition
Lesbian	A woman who is sexually and/or romantically attracted to other women. Some homosexual women will identify as lesbian, others as gay and others as either/both. Some non-binary people may also identify with this term.
LGBTQ+	The umbrella acronym for lesbian, gay, bi, trans, queer, intersex and asexual/aromantic. Other acronyms may be used to similar effect, including 'LGBT', 'LGBT+' and 'LGBTQIA'. 'LGB' as an acronym is sometimes used in research that is specific to minority sexual orientations.
Misgendering	To refer to someone using words or pronouns which do not match with their gender identity. This may be accidental or malicious and purposeful; however, misgendering is offensive and psychologically harmful. See also 'Deadnaming'.
MSM/WSW	MSM (men who have sex with men) and WSW (women who have sex with women) are terms to refer to sexual behaviour only and carry no assumptions about the way in which people identify. These terms are usually utilised in research, public health and policy. Not all MSM or WSW would identify as gay/lesbian/bisexual.
Non-binary/NB/Gender non-conforming	Someone whose gender identity does not comfortably conform to the binary identities of 'man' or 'woman'. Non-binary identities are varied and can include people who identify with some aspects of binary identities, while others reject them entirely. 'Genderqueer' may also be used in this sense.
Outed	When an LGBTQ+ person's sexual orientation or gender identity is disclosed to someone else without their consent. This may be accidental or malicious and purposeful.
Pansexual/Pan	Someone who is sexually and romantically attracted to people of all genders. This term is similar to bisexual but does not imply only two genders.
Pronouns	Words used in place of a name to refer to someone in conversation – for example, 'he' or 'she'. Some people may prefer others to refer to them in gender neutral language and use pronouns such as they/their.
Queer	An umbrella term for anyone who is not heterosexual and cisgender. Queer is also a term used by those wanting to reject specific labels of romantic orientation, sexual orientation and/or gender identity. While it can and is often used as an affirmative and inclusive label, this term has historically been used in a derogatory manner, so caution is advised in its use.
Queerphobia	An umbrella term used to describe the prejudice faced by people of minority sexual orientations and gender identities, a collaboration of the distinct experiences of homophobia, biphobia and transphobia.
Questioning	The process of exploring one's own sexual orientation and/or gender identity.
Sex/Sex assigned at birth	Biologically defined and genetically/hormonally driven characteristics related to physiology and reproductive capabilities of males and females. Typically assigned to a person at birth on the basis of primary sex characteristics, notably external genitalia. See also 'Intersex'.
Sexuality/Sexual orientation	Sexual attraction to other people, or lack thereof. Often linked with 'romantic orientation' to describe someone's sexual and/or romantic attraction to others. Examples include (but are not limited to) homosexual, bisexual and heterosexual.
Spectrum	A term used to cover a variety of identities that have a root commonality or shared experience.
SOGI	Acronym for Sexual Orientation and Gender Identity. Often used in the context of people of minority SOGI.
Transgender/Trans	Someone whose gender identity differs from the sex that they were assigned at birth. Typically, transgender refers to someone whose gender identity is the binary opposite of their sex assigned at birth.
Transgender man/Trans man	Someone who was assigned female at birth but identifies and lives as a man. The term FtM (female to male) may be seen but is a historical term and should be avoided.
Transgender woman/Trans woman	Someone who was assigned male at birth but identifies and lives as a woman. The term MtF (male to female) may be seen but is a historical term and should be avoided.
Transitioning	The process by which some transgender people change their gender expression to align more closely with how they view their gender identity. This may involve social transition (use of different pronouns, dressing and behaving differently) or medical transition (use of hormone therapy +/– surgical interventions). Each trans person's transition is an individual process, and assumptions should not be made about what constitutes 'full' or 'complete' transition.
Transphobia	The dislike of or prejudice specifically against transgender people. This may manifest in intentional misgendering or exclusion.
Transsexual	This is a historical term for what we now call transgender/trans, and should be avoided, but it is worth noting that some trans people may still preferentially use this term.

Adapted from: www.stonewall.org.uk/help-advice/information-and-resources/faqs-and-glossary/list-lgbtq-terms
https://mindout.org.uk/mindouts-lgbtq-glossary
www.who.int/health-topics/gender#tab=tab_1

to) homosexual, which is sexual or romantic attraction to others of one's own gender; bisexual/pansexual, a sexual or romantic attraction to others of multiple genders; and asexual/ aromantic, which is limited or absent sexual or romantic attraction to others (Box 7.1).

Box 7.1 **Alan, 45 years. 'I'm very comfortable being gay. I have a happy life.'**

'I must have been 16 or 17 before I really thought about my sexuality. I'd dated a few girls, but it was only for a short while, and it never lasted long. It always felt a bit off, and I think at the time, I put it down to not being a right match. I had feelings about other boys, but it wasn't something you talked openly about, and I just suppressed it and told myself it was a phase. There were always times when there was "banter", as they say, but it was usually a bit negative. I kissed a couple of boys once or twice, but we put it down to being drunk and didn't talk about it afterwards.

It wasn't really until my early 20s and doing an apprenticeship that I met my first serious boyfriend. It was quite intense, and we became exclusive after a few months; we moved in together. Looking back, it's funny doing all the things like trying to get a mortgage, meeting the in-laws, you know, the usual. Actually, it was painful at times – barriers were put in the way when we were just two people in love like anyone else. There was still a lot of prejudice around.

We broke up after a few years, and I did go through a bad patch; anxiety and drinking too much. I threw myself into the club scene. While it was a tough time, it's also how I met Sam, and now we've been together for 11 years! We got married a year after it became legal, and now honestly, I couldn't be happier. Mind you, even though things have improved a lot, you still have to plan things; you need to know which areas to avoid and so on. I'm still awkward about holding hands or kissing in public in case we get the wrong kind of attention. All in all, I am happy: I have a wonderful husband and a very close group of friends.'

While individuals of minority sexual orientations and gender identities fall within the combined category of LGBTQ+, these are separate and distinct aspects of identity. Someone may be of a minority gender identity while also being heterosexual, while others may be of a minority gender identity and minority sexual orientation simultaneously. Gender identity and sexual orientation are not one and the same. Assumptions should not be made on one aspect of a person's identity based on knowledge of another.

Transgender/non-binary

The most common gender identity is cisgender: those whose gender identity matches their sex assigned at birth – for example, an individual assigned female at birth whose gender identity is a woman. Minority gender identities are transgender and gender non-binary identities. Transgender people are those whose gender identity is one of the binary identities (man or woman), but that gender is different from their sex assigned at birth. An example would be someone assigned female at birth but whose gender identity is that of a man.

Non-binary gender identities are similar to transgender identities as there is a difference between one's gender identity and the sex assigned at birth. The difference, however, is that non-binary gender identities lie outside the binary genders of 'man' and 'woman'. There

is a range of different identities within this umbrella term, from those who are a combination of aspects of 'man' and 'woman', those whose identity is fluid and changes with time, or those who feel an affinity with neither 'man' nor 'woman' but with a third gender entirely (see Further reading/resources)

Transition

Transition is the process by which a person who is transgender or non-binary changes their gender expression to match their true gender identity more closely. This is a deeply personal process and will be a unique and individual journey for each person. Elements of transition are broadly categorised into 'social' and 'medical'. Social transition elements include (but are not limited to) change of name and pronouns, change of gender expression through clothes and mannerisms or use of adjuncts to aid presentation (for example, chest binders to flatten breasts). Medical transition includes the range of available cosmetic, medical and surgical interventions that can support an individual's gender expression. These include (but are not limited to) hair removal procedures, use of feminising or masculinising hormone therapy and gender affirmation surgeries (Box 7.2).

Box 7.2 **Sandra, 34. 'It's been a tough road, and I'm not there yet.'**

'I knew very early on that I wasn't a boy. It's difficult, though; who do you talk to? And what do you say?

I've been in some bad situations. I thought the feelings would pass, but they were difficult to live with. In my mind, I have been Sandra since my early 20s, but it was much more difficult being open about it, even to family and "friends". I tried a relationship with a man, but it ended in violence, and I was in a really bad way. I did anything I could to escape the dysphoria – drink, drugs, even church.

At first, everyone seemed kind and wanted to help, but everything changed when I trusted them enough to tell them what was happening inside me – how I really felt. It soon became about "praying for our brother to be delivered", me changing and not them accepting me as I am.

So now I let myself be who I know I am, at least at home. I'm careful to dress down when I go out though, or I end up receiving abusive comments. I've tried going to the police, but they don't take it seriously. It's helped that so many people use pronouns now. For me, adding my pronouns to my email was a huge help. At first, it was scary, but it's been really liberating to finally say, "Yes, this is who I am! Deal with it!". Actually, a few people at work have been very supportive. There have been times I've been for job interviews, though when I see the reaction on their faces, I know I've lost before I even start.

I'm trying to transition now, but the clinic's waiting list is so long that sometimes I feel like I'll never get there. It can be really isolating, and it would be nice to have more support. There are helpful online support groups, but I live in the country, and there isn't a local trans group.'

It is not required of any transgender or non-binary person to undertake all of the above. Transition is a deeply personal process. There are many reasons why not all the steps above will be a part of someone's transition. While some measures may not be undertaken due to negative reasons – such as stigma or fear of prejudice – this reason should not be assumed. Many trans and non-binary people may have happily completed their transition by social elements of transition alone.

Queer

It is important to be aware of the term 'Queer' and cautious in its use. Historically, queer was used as a derogatory term for LGBTQ+ people, and for many in the community, still bears hurtful associations with experiences of abuse. However, it has recently been reclaimed by many in the LGBTQ+ community as a positive affirmation of an inclusive community. Often, it is used by LGBTQ+ people as a term for anyone who is not cisgendered and heterosexual. It is often used not only as an inclusive label but as a rejection of social norms and expectations concerning sexual orientation and gender identity.

Homophobia/biphobia/transphobia

Experiences of prejudice and discrimination are common among all protected characteristics. While there are common themes, each category of protected characteristic will also experience discrimination unique to them. Experiences of racism will be similar in some ways to experiences of sexism but unique in other ways. Similarly, there is discrimination faced uniquely by the LGBTQ+ community and groups within it. Prejudice and discrimination related to sexual orientation are often termed homophobia. Sometimes discrimination specifically aimed at bisexual people is called biphobia. Likewise, prejudice and discrimination experienced by transgender and non-binary people is called transphobia.

While it is sometimes helpful to put these experiences into subcategories, it is also useful to discuss experiences of prejudice and discrimination faced by the LGBTQ+ community as a whole. This is often referred to as queerphobia or occasionally LGBTphobia. There are many shared root causes of prejudice and discrimination aimed at LGBTQ+ people.

LGBTQ+ health inequalities

All healthcare professionals should understand that while minority sexual orientations and gender identities are not psychiatric conditions, many health inequalities and adverse health outcomes are more prevalent in the LGBTQ+ community. Historically, equal treatment of minoritised people has been considered the desired outcome of Equality, Diversity and Inclusion (EDI) initiatives. However, as the understanding of inequalities faced by minority groups has advanced, this dogma has become outdated. In healthcare, where the aim is holistic treatment of patients as individuals, clinicians should not simply provide equal care to patients with protected characteristics but also address any potential adverse health outcomes.

For LGBTQ+ patients specifically, it is helpful to consider broad themes of health inequalities. Understanding themes of health inequalities provides a deeper appreciation of the underlying causes of these inequalities. This helps clinicians better understand their LGBTQ+ patients. These health inequalities are underresearched. Understanding these health inequalities allows clinicians to appreciate likely health inequalities experienced by their LGBTQ+ patients, which are not yet fully described in contemporary data.

Experiences of healthcare

The experiences of LGBTQ+ people in accessing healthcare may account for many of the health inequalities discussed here. Negative experiences of healthcare provision range from inappropriate comments by healthcare staff to overt attempts to pressure patients into so-called 'conversion therapy' (Box 7.3). In total, 23% of LGBTQ+ people have experienced anti-LGBTQ+ remarks from healthcare staff, rising to 40% in transgender patients [3, 4]. These experiences erode the trust of LGBTQ+ patients in healthcare providers and dissuade them from accessing healthcare. 14% of LGBTQ+ people have avoided treatment due to fear of discrimination, with this figure rising to 37% in transgender people [3].

> **Box 7.3** **Patrick, 51. 'My asthma nurse said to me, "I expect people like you get lots of chest infections".'**
>
> 'I grew up in a strict Irish Catholic family, so it was complete rejection when I finally plucked up the courage to come out as gay. Practically driven out of the family, I was. My brother kept in touch with me, and he and his wife have been fantastic over the years. Always invite me for Christmas, provided my parents weren't visiting …
>
> My family have always been big drinkers, and the rejection has always been hard for me. So, I drink more than I probably should. I think I need a good doctor, but they are difficult to find in my experience. I've registered at a few different GPs after some bad experiences, and I just don't think I can talk about my family issues any more.
>
> I've got a lot of problems with asthma, so I need prescriptions and check-ups, you know. I hate having to go there. They're bigots, all of them. I was in for my flu jab last year with the nurse. She was perfectly pleasant, but she said, "And don't get carried away partying over Christmas. I know what you lot are like".
>
> I've been in a stable relationship for years, married now even. When I walk into the GP surgery waiting room with my husband, I just feel unwelcome and the knowing looks between them all.'

LGBTQ+ patients report a lack of specific understanding of their healthcare needs from healthcare providers; 25% of LGBTQ+ people reported a lack of specific healthcare needs relating to their sexuality by healthcare providers, with this figure rising to 62% in transgender people [3].

Mental health

While minority sexual orientations and gender identities are neither mental health nor psychiatric conditions, there are significant mental health problems associated with the experiences of LGBTQ+ individuals. Levels of anxiety and depression are significantly higher in the LGBTQ+ community than in the general population (Figures 7.1 and 7.2).

These poor mental health trends are sadly significantly worse when considering transgender and gender non-binary people specifically; 46% of transgender people report having considered suicide in the last year alone, compared with 31% of cisgender LGB people [3]. Sadly, numbers of those who attempted suicide are higher also, with 12% of transgender people in the last year alone, compared with 2% of cisgender LGB people. These trends are distressing but predictable when considering the degree of psychological stress created by societal prejudice combined with reduced willingness to access support from healthcare.

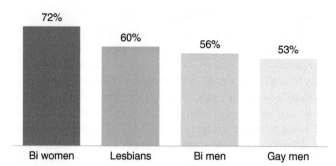

Figure 7.1 Percentage of LGBQT+ people who report anxiety in the preceding year. Data adapted from 'LGBT in Britain – Health Report', Stonewall 2018 [3].

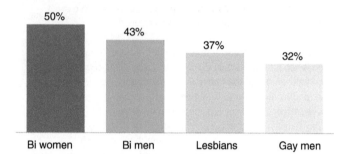

Figure 7.2 Percentage of LGBQT+ people reporting their life was not worth living in the past year. Data adapted from 'LGBT in Britain – Health Report', Stonewall 2018 [3].

Substance misuse

Rates of smoking, alcohol use and use of illicit drugs are all higher in the LGBTQ+ community. Rates of tobacco smoking in LGBTQ+ people are significantly higher by comparison with the general population (Figure 7.3). Specific, contemporary data for rates of tobacco use in transgender and gender non-binary people are unknown. Alcohol use is also higher within the LGBTQ+ community, with daily alcohol consumption reported in 16% of LGBTQ+ people compared to 10% in the general population [3]. This rises with age and 33% of LGBTQ+ people over 65 report daily alcohol consumption [3]. This trend continues with substance misuse, with 28.4% of LGBTQ+ people having taken illicit substances in the previous year compared with 8.1% of the general population [5].

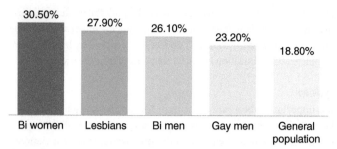

Figure 7.3 Percentage of LGBTQ+ who are tobacco smokers compared to the general population. Data adapted from 'The odds of smoking by sexual orientation in England', 2016 [6].

These trends are not unpredictable. Historically, safe spaces for the LGBTQ+ community have always been bars. Gay bars and later LGBTQ+ venues have long been home to the LGBTQ+ community. So it is unsurprising that many LGBTQ+ people have formed associations between the use of alcohol, tobacco and even illicit substances and feelings of safety, community and belonging.

Physical health

The majority of health inequalities faced by the LGBTQ+ communities are those described above. There are also important (and often unexpected) physical health inequalities. Data are lacking concerning prevalence and outcomes for most general physical health among the LGBTQ+ population. The available data relate mainly to the uptake of screening programmes and sexual health. 15% of lesbian and bisexual women have never had a cervical smear test, compared with 7% of women in the general population [7]. Transgender people are often failed by automated systems, which – when gender markers are changed on digital systems – cease to continue sending invitations for appropriate screening appointments.

The topic of sexual health in the LGBTQ+ community is vast and well researched in contrast to other LGBTQ+ health inequalities. A comprehensive breakdown of sexual health inequalities experienced by the LGBTQ+ community is outside this chapter's scope. It is worth noting, however, that new STI diagnoses in gay and bisexual men have seen significant increases in recent years (Figure 7.4), while less than half of lesbian and bisexual women have ever undergone an STI screen [8].

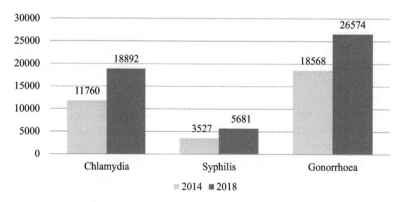

Figure 7.4 Increase in new STI diagnoses in gay men, bisexual men and men who have sex with men between 2014 and 2018. Data taken from 'Sexually transmitted infections and screening for chlamydia in England', 2018 [7].

Social health

The social experiences of LGBTQ+ people interact closely with their health. Clinicians should understand the impact of this. The landscape of prejudice, discrimination and abuse faced by the LGBTQ+ community significantly affects health; 40% of LGBTQ+ people report having experienced negative incidents in the previous year about their sexual orientation or gender identity, including verbal harassment, threats of physical violence and direct experience of physical or sexual violence [4]. Furthermore, 18% of LGBTQ+ people have been homeless at some point in their lives, with 24% of homeless young people identifying as LGBTQ+ [9,10].

LGBTQ+ people are also more likely to have experienced domestic abuse, with 11% of LGBTQ+ people in the previous year compared with 6% of women and 3% of men in the general population [9]. This is more prevalent in transgender and non-binary people, 19% of whom have experienced domestic abuse in the last year alone [9].

Loneliness and isolation are higher in the LGBTQ+ community, particularly when considering older LGBTQ+ people. Forty-one percent of LGB people live alone compared to 28% of heterosexual people, and 50% of LGB people over 50 report feelings of isolation [11].

Queerphobia in the NHS

Alongside negative experiences of LGBTQ+ people in healthcare, there is also the impact of queerphobia within the health service itself. A survey in 2016 of doctors and medical students reported that more than 70% of respondents had experienced homophobic or biphobic harassment or abuse at their place of work or study within the last two years [12]. Concerningly, only a quarter of those affected had reported the incident [12]. These findings regarding the prevalence of prejudiced views within the modern-day health service are concerning (Boxes 7.4 and 7.5). An updated survey is pending in 2023.

Box 7.4 Nisha, 25. 'Well, at least you won't have to worry about choosing between kids and a career.'

'I'm hoping to stay in hospital medicine though I'm not sure which specialty yet. Surgery maybe?

I love the team spirit in hospitals, especially in acute areas like MAU and A&E. I've not particularly mentioned my sexuality, but I get many offers from men. I usually just say I'm already with someone, and if they push, I'll say my girlfriend. I once had a comment from a doctor saying that I was letting all my talent go to waste on a girlfriend. I tried to change the subject, but he carried on and asked me out, saying that he could show me a "good time" and "turn me straight again". It was so upsetting, and I was absolutely livid. I couldn't bring myself to make a complaint though – not because I thought it was acceptable but because somehow, I'd be seen as the troublemaker. So, I just bit my tongue whenever we were on shift together until I moved jobs.

There is still homophobia out there in the NHS. Sometimes, staff make jokes about some of the patients when they are on break, especially the same-sex couples, or they say it's not normal. It's awful, but at least people will come and have a quiet word about it, you know, to check I'm ok.'

Box 7.5 Robbie, 37. 'I think I should have changed jobs when I transitioned.'

'I was already working in a senior role when I started my transition. I'd reached a plateau in my career; my partner and family were supportive. So, the time seemed right.

I did think about changing jobs at the time or taking some time out, but I'd always felt supported by my team at work, and they knew about some of my life outside medicine. We had all done the annual Equality, Diversity and Inclusion training together, and I thought the conversation was always very empathetic towards LGBTQ+ staff and patients.

Things did seem to change once I began to be open about my plans and changed my pronouns. There were comments about my adding to everyone's workload while I went off for treatment. Apparently, some people still refer to me as "she" when I'm not there. A patient said she had told one of my team I was a very nice man, and my colleague said, "Yes, well, he's not a real man, of course". That was really hurtful to hear.

It's disappointing in a caring profession, particularly as I've had no clinical performance issues. The worst part is the performative support – some of the people who wear rainbow lanyards are the ones who say this stuff behind my back.'

Practising allyship

While it is essential to understand the experience of LGBTQ+ communities, it is of arguably greater importance for healthcare staff to practise good allyship for their colleagues and advocacy for their patients (see also Chapter 12). Primarily, clinicians should avoid assumptions. Assumptions regarding the gender of people's partners or correct pronouns can lead to avoidable distress. If there is uncertainty about this information, a sensitively worded question will probably help the situation. The patient or colleague will likely feel validated by the interest. Where mistakes are made, a sensitive and genuine apology will often adequately remedy any offence caused. Such an apology must be accompanied by efforts to amend, i.e. using correct pronouns after being informed. Training should be provided to clinicians on skills such as inclusive history taking (Box 7.6).

Box 7.6 Inclusive history-taking.

- Ask open-ended questions. Follow the patient's lead.
- Be respectful and non-judgemental.
- Make no assumptions.
  - Do not assume you know the patient's gender identity.
  - Do not assume you know the patient's sexual orientation.
  - Do not assume that patients' reported relationship status defines their choice of partners.
  - Do not assume that patients' sexual orientations determine whether they want to parent a child.
  - Do not assume that patients' sexual orientation determines whether they may be affected by domestic/relationship violence.
- When you don't know, ask.

Source: https://sites.tufts.edu/tuftsbqa/files/2016/04/BQA-Curriculum-Recs-2018.pdf (accessed 30th July 2022).

While daunting, particularly in healthcare systems wherein hierarchies persist, healthcare staff must challenge queerphobic behaviour. This is encouraged if it can safely be done directly and in the moment (see Chapter 12). However, it cannot always be done safely. If this is the case, alternative ways exist to escalate such concerns within departments and institutions' Human Resources departments. Ultimately, if someone is the victim of prejudicial remarks, the practice of good allyship would include checking in with that person afterwards and offering support in escalating concerns via appropriate channels.

There are specific issues about supporting transgender and non-binary patients. Occasionally, it is important for the medical care of a transgender or non-binary patient to know specific details that would be inappropriate to enquire about in non-medical settings. These include issues relating to the use of hormone replacement therapy and any changes to internal or external anatomy. An example of this is if a trans man presents with abdominal pain. In this case, it is clinically extremely important to know whether this patient still has a uterus and ovaries, and clinicians should ask this. How the question is asked, however, is vitally important. If it is unclear why this question is being asked, the patient may think that the clinician is being unnecessarily curious about unrelated issues. Likewise, if it is not clinically relevant to know these details, then do not ask.

Healthcare professionals should be cautious not to disclose information about LGBTQ+ patients and colleagues without their permission. However, this can be inadvertent. Healthcare professionals should exercise caution, particularly when calling patients from waiting rooms or if information about their sexuality or gender identity is not yet known to family members. Such disclosures can profoundly damage the professional's trust with patients and colleagues.

Conclusion

The LGBTQ+ community continues to face significant challenges with respect to healthcare, including a range of health inequalities damaging their physical, mental and social health and wellbeing. Healthcare professionals should understand the breadth and diversity of this community. While the extent of terminology can be daunting at first, a comprehensive understanding of key concepts regarding sexuality and gender identity will improve the holistic care of LGBTQ+ patients.

Further reading/resources

General information

Stonewall. www.stonewall.org.uk/help-advice/information-and-resources (accessed 30th September 2022)

Being gay is okay. https://bgiok.org.uk (accessed 30th September 2022).

British Medical Association, GLADD The Association of LGBTQ+ Doctors and Dentists (2022). Sexual Orientation and Gender Identity in the Medical Profession. https://www.bma.org.uk/media/6340/bma-sogi-report-2-nov-2022.pdf. (accessed 18 February 2023)

Healthcare resources

RCGP LGBT Health Hub. https://elearning.rcgp.org.uk/course/index.php (accessed 30th September 2022)

Gender Identity Research and Education Society (GIRES). www.gires.org.uk/category/health (accessed 30th September 2022)

Age UK LGBT+ Health and Wellbeing. www.ageuk.org.uk/information-advice/health-wellbeing/relationships-family/lgbt (accessed 30th September 2022)

National LGB&T Partnership. www.consortium.lgbt/nationallgbtpartnership/publications (accessed 30th September 2022)

Vincent, B. (2018) *Transgender Health: A Practitioner's Guide to Binary and Non-Binary Trans Patient Care*. London: Jessica Kingsley Publishers.

Vincent, B. (2020) *Non-binary Genders: Navigating Communities, Identities, and Healthcare*. London: Policy Press.

Reports on health inequalities

Government Equalities Office National LGBT Survey. www.gov.uk/government/publications/national-lgbt-survey-summary-report (accessed 30th September 2022)

References

1 Public Health England (2017). Producing Modelled Estimates of the Size of the Lesbian, Gay and Bisexual (LGB) Population of England. https://assets.publishing.service.gov.uk/government/uploads/system/uploads/attachment_data/file/585349/PHE_Final_report_FINAL_DRAFT_14.12.2016NB230117v2.pdf (accessed 30 September 2022)

2 Gender Identity Research and Education Society (GIRES) (2015) Monitoring Gender Nonconformity – A Quick Guide. www.gires.org.uk/wp-content/uploads/2014/09/Monitoring-Gender-Nonconformity.pdf (accessed 30 September 2022)

3 Bachmann, C. and Gooch, B. (2018) LGBT in Britain. Health Report. www.stonewall.org.uk/system/files/lgbt_in_britain_health.pdf (accessed 30 September 2022)

4 Government Equalities Office (2018) LGBT Survey Summary Report. https://assets.publishing.service.gov.uk/government/uploads/system/uploads/attachment_data/file/722314/GEO-LGBT-Survey-Report.pdf (accessed 30 September 2022)

5 Home Office (2014) Drug Misuse: Findings from the 2013/14 Crime Survey for England and Wales. www.gov.uk/government/statistics/drug-misuse-findings-from-the-2013-to-2014-csew/drug-misuse-findings-from-the-201314-crime-survey-for-england-and-wales#estimates-of-illicit-drug-use-by-ethnicity-and-sexual-orientation (accessed 30 September 2022)

6 Office for National Statistics (2018) The odds of smoking by sexual orientation in England. www.ons.gov.uk/peoplepopulationandcommunity/healthandsocialcare/healthinequalities/adhocs/009373theoddsofsmokingbysexualorientationinengland2016#:~:text=Thegapinsmokingprevalencebetweenheterosexualandgay%2Flesbian,%25CI1.19-1.59 (accessed 30 September 2022)

7 Public Health England (2018) Sexually Transmitted Infections and Screening for Chlamydia in England, 2018. https://pcwhf.co.uk/wp-content/uploads/2019/06/hpr1919_stis-ncsp_ann18.pdf (accessed 30 September 2022)

8 Backmann, C. and Gooch, B. (2018) LGBT in Britain. Home and Communities Report. www.stonewall.org.uk/sites/default/files/lgbt_in_britain_home_and_communities.pdf (accessed 30 September 2022)

9 Albert Kennedy Trust (2015) LGBT Youth Homelessness: A UK National Scoping of Cause, Prevalence, Response, and Outcome. www.akt.org.uk/Handlers/Download.ashx?IDMF=c0f29272-512a-45e8-9f9b-0b76e477baf1.

10 LGBT Foundation (2020) Hidden Figures: LGBT Health Inequalities in the UK. https://lgbt.foundation/hiddenfigures (accessed 30 September 2022)

11 British Medical Association. GLADD – The Association of LGBTQ+ Doctors and Dentists (2016) The Experience of Lesbian, Gay and Bisexual Doctors in the NHS. www.bma.org.uk/media/4225/bma_experience-of-lgb-doctors-and-medical-students-in-nhs-2016.pdf (accessed 30 September 2022)

12 Hunt, R. and Fish, J. (2008) Prescription for Change. Lesbian and Bisexual Women's Health Check. www.stonewall.org.uk/resources/prescription-change-2008 (accessed 30 September 2022)

CHAPTER 8

Disability Disparities and Ableism in Medicine

Lisa I. Iezzoni

Professor of Medicine, Health Policy Research Center, Mongan Institute, Massachusetts General Hospital; Department of Medicine, Harvard Medical School, Boston, USA

OVERVIEW

- Disability is part of the human condition. Almost all of us will face some impairment at some stage of our lives.
- Many disabled people are disadvantaged in social determinants of health.
- People with disabilities experience worse communication with their healthcare professionals, particularly around explanations for their health conditions.
- Patients with disabilities experience diagnostic overshadowing when new symptoms are attributed to the patient's pre-existing disability.
- Multiple barriers exist in healthcare settings for patients with disabilities.
- Healthcare professionals should be trained in basic competencies related to disability.

Introduction

More than 1 billion people globally, about 15% of the world's population, have some type of disability [1]. As defined by the World Health Organization (Box 8.1), disabilities are diverse. They can be congenital, occur suddenly or progress over time. Disabilities can involve mobility, vision, hearing, communication, intellect, learning, thinking, memory, mental health or chronic health conditions, and some people have multiple disabilities.

'Disability is part of the human condition. Almost everyone will be temporarily or permanently impaired at some point in life, and those who survive to old age will experience increasing difficulties in functioning.' [1]

Box 8.1 Definition of disability.

Disability is an 'umbrella term for impairments, activity limitations or participation restrictions', conceiving 'a person's functioning and disability … as a dynamic interaction between health conditions (diseases, disorders, injuries, traumas, etc.) and contextual factors', including social, attitudinal and physical environments and personal characteristics.

Source: World Health Organization [1], p.3.

Despite this near universality across the lifespan, disability remains frequently stigmatised, and disabled people confront barriers to full participation in daily activities and community life. Many people with disabilities are disadvantaged in social determinants of health, including poverty, unemployment, low education, substandard housing and inadequate transportation. Furthermore, worldwide, 'health services are often lower quality, not affordable, and inaccessible for people with disabilities … People with disabilities face higher healthcare needs, more barriers to accessing services, and less health coverage, resulting in worse outcomes' [2].

This chapter provides an overview of several critical health and healthcare considerations for people with disabilities. At the outset, it is important to emphasise that language choices affect perceptions of disability [3]. For example, 'cripple' conveys pity and shame; calling people by their impairment (e.g. 'the quadriplegic', 'the schizophrenic') is degrading. Several decades ago, person-first language – leading with personhood, followed by disability (i.e. 'person with a disability') – took hold, especially in the US. In recent years, communities claiming and celebrating their disability identity have flipped this word order, placing their disability identity first (i.e. 'disabled person'). A November 2019–January 2020 British Medical Association (BMA) survey of 705 disabled doctors and medical students used identity-first language because it reflected the preferences of most participants [4].

Nevertheless, some people with disabling conditions do not view themselves as disabled for personal, cultural or other reasons. In the 2020 BMA survey (p.7), 90% of participants indicated they had a condition covered under the Equality Act 2010 definition of disability, but only 48% considered themselves disabled. Certain communities explicitly eschew this label. For instance, sign language users often see themselves as a linguistic or cultural minority, signalling this identity by spelling Deaf with a capital D. Some individuals who are autistic, dyslexic or otherwise neurodivergent identify as disabled, while others do not. Thus, language choices are evolving, complex and vary by individual preferences. Recognising these differing views, this chapter alternates between person-first and identity-first language. Healthcare professionals must understand and honour patients' disability-related language preferences to convey respect and build trust.

ABC of Equality, Diversity and Inclusion in Healthcare, First Edition. Edited by Shehla Imtiaz-Umer and John Frain.
© 2023 John Wiley & Sons Ltd. Published 2023 by John Wiley & Sons Ltd.

Brief disability history

Early human societies – hunter-gatherers – recognised that some people could neither hunt nor gather and needed assistance to survive. Nonetheless, from early times, questions arose about who deserved societal support. The Old Testament Book of Leviticus (21:16) enumerated 'blemishes' that precluded people from 'drawing near' during religious ceremonies: 'a man blind or lame, or one who has a mutilated face or a limb too long ... or a hunchback, or a dwarf ... ' In the Middle Ages, clergy warned that God punished moral failings by inflicting disability upon parishioners. Determining which individuals with disability merited support posed problems. In fourteenth-century Europe, local authorities determined that some supplicants were lazy, malingering or faking disability to avoid labour and receive food, housing or other subsistence. Therefore, 'the concept of disability has always been based on a perceived need to detect deception' (Stone, 1984 – see Further reading).

In the nineteenth century, rapid innovations in medical diagnostic technologies (e.g. stethoscope, microscope, ophthalmoscope, radiograph) offered putatively objective means to identify disease and thus validate disability. These new tools also shifted perceptions of disability from supernatural visitations to biological causes. Wielding these technologies, physicians attained the authority to determine disability and thus who deserved disability-related societal benefits (Stone, 1984 – see Further reading). This generated the medical model of disability (Box 8.2), which views disability as an individual circumstance that persons should overcome or mitigate under medical intervention or guidance. If cure or improvement remains unattainable, the medical model expects people to adapt and accept their limitations.

Box 8.2 **Medical model of disability.**

'The *medical model* views disability as a problem of the person, directly caused by disease, trauma, or other health condition, which requires medical care ... Management of the disability is aimed at cure or the individual's adjustment and behaviour change. Medical care is viewed as the main issue ... '

Source: World Health Organization [1], p.20.

Accelerating in the 1970s, disability rights advocates pushed back against the medical model and authority of healthcare professionals. The independent living movement rejected the notion that needing assistance to perform even basic activities of daily living (ADLs: feeding, bathing, dressing, toileting, basic mobility) represents dependency. Instead, advocates argued that disability is not a problem of individuals but of social and physical environments that fail to accommodate functional impairments. Barriers are 'imposed on top of our impairments by the way we are unnecessarily isolated and excluded from full participation in society' (Olkin, 1999, p. 22 – see Further reading). Gaining agency from these views, an activated disability community aimed to overcome these barriers. These attitudes coalesced into the social model of disability (Box 8.3), which positioned disability as a human rights issue.

Box 8.3 **Social model of disability.**

'The *social model* ... sees the issue mainly as a socially created problem, and basically as a matter of the full integration of individuals into society. Disability is not an attribute of an individual but rather a complex collection of conditions, many of which are created by the social environment ... The issue is, therefore, an attitudinal or ideological one requiring social change, which at the political level becomes a question of human rights.'

Source: World Health Organization [1], p.20.

Since then, countries worldwide have enacted laws protecting the civil rights of people with disabilities, including mandating equitable healthcare. Adopted by the United Nations General Assembly in 2006, the Convention on the Rights of Persons with Disabilities (CRPD) eight guiding principles (Box 8.4) underscore its social justice perspective. CRPD Article 25, Health, requires proactive initiatives to ensure equal quality healthcare for disabled people. Despite rejection by disability communities, however, the medical model and discriminatory ableist attitudes persist in many healthcare settings.

Box 8.4 **United Nations Convention on the Rights of Persons with Disabilities: guiding principles.**

1 Respect for inherent dignity, individual autonomy, including the freedom to make one's own choices, and independence of persons
2 Non-discrimination
3 Full and effective participation and inclusion in society
4 Respect for difference and acceptance of persons with disabilities as part of human diversity and humanity
5 Equality of opportunity
6 Accessibility
7 Equality between men and women
8 Respect for the evolving capacities of children with disabilities and respect for the right of children with disabilities to preserve their identities

---

Healthcare disparities for people with disability

Worldwide, people with disability experience disparities in their healthcare and worse health outcomes. However, the extent and nature of disparities vary by disability type, patients' sociodemographic characteristics, geographic location (e.g. urban versus rural) and specific health care service. For instance, in 2010–2018, 83.0% of non-disabled US women aged 30 years and older reported having had a mammogram in the last two years compared with 71.4% of women with complex activity limitations [5]. Also, in the US, women with disability and early-stage breast cancer had lower relative risks of obtaining breast-conserving surgery (0.80 [95% confidence interval 0.76–0.84]) versus mastectomy; among those undergoing breast-conserving surgery, women with disability had lower adjusted relative risks of radiotherapy (0.83 [0.77–0.90]) and axillary node dissection (0.81 [0.74–0.90]) (McCarthy et al., 2006 – see Further reading). For early-stage breast cancer, women with mental disorders or neurological conditions were much less likely to have breast-conserving surgery than women with cardiorespiratory or musculoskeletal disorders (Iezzoni et al., 2008 – see Further reading). Women with disability had higher rates of all-cause mortality and breast cancer-specific mortality than non-disabled women (McCarthy et al., 2007 – see Further reading). Most troubling, women with pre-existing disability have a higher adjusted odds of being diagnosed with breast cancer (1.21, p = 0.04) compared to non-disabled women [5].

Disparities occur across the healthcare delivery system, although the absence of routine disability data collection hampers the identification and monitoring of these inequities. Compared with non-disabled patients, for example, Americans with disabilities generally report worse communication with their clinicians, especially not receiving clear explanations about their health conditions and not understanding the next steps for their care [6]. Patients with hearing loss report that some physicians communicate through note writing, lip reading, talking more slowly or shouting rather than by providing communication accommodations; communication problems decrease patients' adherence and trust in their clinicians [7]. Failure to provide sign language interpreters for Deaf patients can also cause anxiety and fear (Box 8.5) (Iezzoni et al., 2004 – see Further reading). Some physicians erroneously believe that patients with disability are sexually inactive and thus at low risk of human papillomavirus exposure, justifying not recommending cervical cancer screening (Chen et al., 2009 – see Further reading). As for breast cancer, compared to their non-disabled peers, women with pre-existing disability have a higher adjusted odds of cervical cancer (1.43, p = 0.03); nevertheless, in the US, only 67.6% of women with chronic mobility limitations aged 18 and older reported Pap (cervical) smears within the prior three years, compared with 81.0% of non-disabled women [5].

Box 8.5 **Communication failures.**

Alison and Harry were born deaf; they speak sign language. Each asked for a sign language interpreter for their primary care visits. Their physicians refused, saying that Alison and Harry were young and healthy, the visits were routine, and a sign language interpreter was therefore not necessary.

Alison's first Pap test (cervical smear)
'They didn't tell me what they were going to do. There I was in the stirrups – I couldn't see what was going on. The doctor didn't say to me, "This might be uncomfortable" or tell me how much pain to expect. I never went again.'

Harry's first testicular exam
'I was scared. I didn't know if I was being molested or raped or if this was a sexual advance. A hearing doctor with a hearing patient will talk through the entire exam, but when the patient is deaf, they just do it. Some doctors keep on talking. They forget I'm deaf.'

People with disabilities can also experience diagnostic overshadowing when clinicians erroneously attribute all new signs or symptoms to their underlying disability, thus delaying diagnosis of other, often treatable conditions. Diagnostic overshadowing was first described among persons with intellectual disability and subsequently for persons with serious mental illness [8]. People with other disabilities also experience diagnostic overshadowing. For example, Katie, a young woman with spinal cord injury (SCI), began vomiting, losing weight and having severe abdominal pain [9]. She visited the emergency department five times, and during each encounter, physicians erroneously diagnosed gastroparesis related to her SCI (Box 8.6). Katie's weight loss became life-threatening before physicians finally made the correct diagnosis.

Box 8.6 **Diagnostic overshadowing: young woman with spinal cord injury.**

Katie, 26 years old, had a spinal cord injury (SCI) from a diving accident in her late teens, was paraplegic and used a wheelchair. Five years after the SCI, she developed severe abdominal pain, vomiting and weight loss. Over two years, she repeatedly visited outpatient doctors, who did not weigh her; some asked if she was anorexic or bulimic. She went to the emergency department at a major academic medical center five times, and each time, physicians said she had gastroparesis because of the SCI.

'They said that my stomach, because of the injury, was digesting food slower and that that was the issue. This went on for two years. I was throwing up non-stop. I would wake up and just vomit bile. I couldn't eat. I had no appetite. You could give me my favorite foods, and I would just not even want them … I did tons of research on things to do, and I changed my entire diet. I tried to go vegan, but nothing worked.'

After another emergency department visit, a gastroenterologist finally tested Katie for gastroparesis using a wireless motility capsule (also known as a SmartPill®). The test was negative (i.e. did not show gastroparesis). At that point, Katie's weight loss had become life-threatening: she is 5'11" tall and weighed 68 pounds. Physicians placed a feeding tube under radiographic guidance and found a mass in her lung, later diagnosed as Hodgkin lymphoma.

Barriers to care for people with disability

Multiple barriers impede access to care for disabled patients, ranging from attitudes and knowledge of healthcare professionals to physical and communication barriers in clinical settings (Table 8.1). In a 2019–2020 survey of US physicians caring for disabled adults in outpatient settings, 35.0% reported that lack of formal education or training was a large or moderate barrier to caring for patients with disability [10]. Only 40.7% of physicians were very confident that they could provide the same quality care to patients with disability as to their non-disabled patients, and just 56.5% strongly agreed that they welcomed disabled patients in their practices [11]. Policies and practices within healthcare delivery systems can exacerbate these concerns. For instance, the US physician survey found that 44.7% of physicians felt that lack of time was a large or moderate barrier to caring for disabled patients [10].

Inaccessible equipment – such as roll-on weight scales or examination tables that do not automatically raise or lower – contributes to disparities and substandard care for patients with mobility disabilities. Clinicians sometimes examine these patients in their wheelchairs,

Table 8.1 Barriers to care for people with disability and recommendations for improving access.

Barriers to care	Recommendations
Ableist and discriminatory attitudes among health care professionals	• Recognize and address implicit and explicit biases and discriminatory attitudes among health care professionals concerning people with disability • Recognize disabled patients as experiencing health and health care disparities • Train health care professionals in disability cultural competence
Inadequate knowledge about caring for disabling conditions and insufficient scientific evidence base	• Include disability topics in healthcare professional training • Include people with disability in clinical trials • Include disability status when collecting routine data used for observational studies
Erroneous assumptions among healthcare professionals about people with disability	• Do not make assumptions about the values or preferences of people with disability; recognise that they value and find pleasure in their lives, as do other people • Recognise that patients with disability may know more about their underlying disabling condition than do their clinicians • Involve patients with disability in collaborative care, shared decision making
Diagnostic overshadowing	• Do not assume that all new signs and symptoms relate to the patient's underlying disabling condition • Perform appropriate diagnostic evaluations of new signs and symptoms to determine the cause accurately • Treat new conditions as appropriate and consistent with the patient's preferences
Failure of clinicians to understand local legal obligations to ensure equitable and accessible care for people with disability	• Understand local laws about ensuring equitable and accessible care to disabled patients • Train clinicians and other staff in providing reasonable accommodations to ensure accessible care • Review and modify policies in practice setting to ensure equitable and accessible care for patients
Barriers to physical access to medical diagnostic equipment and other facilities for patients with physical disability	• Height-adjustable examination table, with accessible stirrups for performing Pap smear, pelvic exams • Wheelchair-accessible weight scale • Accessible diagnostic imaging equipment • Accessible transfer devices • Personal assistance with positioning, dressing/undressing as preferred by disabled patient
Barriers to communication with patients with vision and/or hearing impairments	• Ensure patients with visual impairments receive written materials in accessible format • As preferred by patient, sighted guide to navigate clinical setting, verbally describe setting • Accommodate qualified service animal • In-person or remote sign language interpreter, CART (Communication Access Realtime Transcription) reporter, and/or voice amplification device depending on patient's preference • Masks with clear windows for lip reading, interpreting facial expressions • Closed caption, audio described video educational materials
Ineffective communication in context of patients with comprehension difficulties, mental illness, intellectual disability	• Understand and aim to meet communication needs and preferences of individual patients • Schedule extra time for visit • Use pictorial representations, models or dolls, simple language • Introduce patient to care setting, demonstrate procedure (e.g. mammogram) • Involve trusted caregiver after assessing their trustworthiness

even when complete physical examinations are medically indicated, or do not provide routine services, such as weight measurement or Pap smears [12,13]. Her outpatient doctors never weighed Katie, for example, although weight loss was her most life-threatening problem (Box 8.6). Most US physicians do not use accessible equipment in their outpatient practices. The 2019–2020 US survey found that only 22.6% of physicians reported always or usually using accessible weight scales for people with significant mobility limitations, and 40.3% always or usually used accessible exam tables or chairs [14]. Among participants, 81.3% indicated that lack of funds to purchase accessible equipment posed problems, while 69.5% complained about inadequate space. Although height-adjustable exam tables can cost more than twice as much as fixed-height tables, installing accessible equipment provides important benefits to nursing or other practice staff, including reducing back injuries and injury-associated costs (Fragala, 2016 – see Further reading).

Laws prohibiting discrimination against patients with disabilities have not prevented disparities in their care. One explanation may involve clinicians' lack of awareness or understanding of these laws. The US survey of outpatient physicians found that 35.8% reported knowing little or nothing about their legal responsibilities under the 1990 Americans with Disabilities Act, which covers all healthcare providers and requires equity for disabled patients [15]. Furthermore, 71.2% reported an incorrect understanding of who determines reasonable accommodations during healthcare encounters for patients with disability (decisions require collaboration between patients and providers).

Finally, according to the US survey, 82.4% of outpatient physicians reported that people with significant disability have worse quality of life than non-disabled people [11]. These ableist attitudes may contribute to disparities or substandard care, such as worse quality treatment for cancer [10]. A study involving in-depth interviews with people with severe mobility disability who subsequently developed cancer found that physicians often did not take patients' complaints seriously, attributing them to depression rather than a new underlying disease [9]. One woman described complaining of abdominal pain and fatigue for two years before her uterine cancer was diagnosed. Her doctors had kept telling her, 'Oh, you're just depressed'.

Representation of disabled people in healthcare professions

A healthcare workforce that represents the diversity of the communities it serves offers one potential strategy for addressing healthcare disparities and improving care (Cohen et al., 2002 – see Further reading). Shared lived experiences presumably forestall erroneous assumptions, bolster empathy and enhance cultural competence when physicians and patients come from the same marginalised group. Whether this concordance on key traits, such as gender or race, enhances communication and patients' healthcare experiences is unclear, with research yielding contradictory results (Shen et al., 2018; Takeshita et al., 2020 – see Further reading). Having a diverse healthcare workforce nevertheless has intrinsic societal value.

However, proportionally few physicians identify as disabled. For example, a 2019 national survey of US practising physicians found that only 3.1% (95% CI, 2.6–3.5%) self-identified as having disability [16]. In contrast, 26.7% of US residents aged 18 and older had disabilities in 2019 (Centers for Disease Control and Prevention, 2022 – see Further reading). Multiple barriers have long prevented people with disability from becoming physicians. The ultimate impediment is skepticism about whether disabled people can safely practise medicine [17].

This issue is frequently framed as weighing individual autonomy against public health (Altchuler, 2009 – see Further reading). 'Codes of medical ethics have emphasized the primacy of patient well-being since the time of Hippocrates, particularly when patient needs are in conflict with those of the physician' (Melnick, 2011 – see Further reading). Disability civil rights laws require the provision of reasonable accommodations both to medical students and practising physicians with disability. However, supervisors or educators with little experience in disability accommodation may not fully understand the iterative process required to identify accommodations that effectively support the competent performance of clinical tasks [18].

Countries approach the inclusion of disabled students in medical training in different ways. In the UK, the General Medical Council provides nationwide guidance to all medical schools on approaches to support trainees with disability, albeit recognizing that 'patient safety is the first priority' [19]. The GMC states, 'As the professional regulator, we firmly believe disabled people should be welcomed to the profession and valued for their contributions to patient care'. It asserts that no health condition or disability automatically disqualifies individuals from safely practising medicine. The GMC recommends that training programmes use a case management model, with various professionals working collaboratively to support disabled trainees, including by ensuring accessible environments and appropriate assistive technologies. All UK medical students must meet the same competence standards, called 'Outcomes for Graduates'. During assessments of these outcomes, students can use reasonable adjustments (i.e. accommodations) unless 'the method of performance is part of the competence to be attained' (GMC, 2019 – see Further

reading). However, in the BMA survey of disabled physicians and medical students, only 55% of respondents who reported needing adjustments said they had obtained them (BMA, 2020 – see Further reading). Box 8.7 presents selected comments from BMA survey participants.

Box 8.7 Selected comments from BMA survey of medical students, other trainees and doctors: November 2019-January 2020 [4].

Medical students and other trainees

- 'People often don't understand how chronic illness affects your life and how debilitating it can be at times. While my school supports me, my peers often think I am exaggerating or not telling the truth as they cannot see the pain, I am in.'
- 'The first instinct of my educational supervisor was to tell me that she was worried I would not be able to cope/function as a consultant. She didn't say why or how she thought I would have difficulty, or suggest any ways of helping me, or any changes to my work patterns; she was just letting me know I was unworthy.'
- 'I found occupational health very understanding and supportive, but my trainers were not willing to permit any adjustments. They would not even talk to me about it. They told me I didn't appear to them to be having enough of a problem.'
- 'Great support from occupational health and the consultant in charge of department and supervisor on this job. However, my peers/other juniors often make comments like "You're so lucky you have a day off/don't work nights" or "Wow, how did you swindle that rota?".'
- 'My reasonable adjustments were refused by my medical school as unreasonable despite being contained in OH reports and not involving any cost to the university. They were recommended by the disability service, and then I was sat down with the medical school administration, and they essentially went down the list saying "this won't happen".'

Doctors

- 'One place of work was extremely supportive. I worked there when I was diagnosed. I was keen specifically not to be treated any differently and to keep information very limited in terms of who was aware. They were extremely supportive in respecting this. Also noted that they were prepared to "bend over backwards" if there was something they could help with.'
- 'After I disclosed my medical condition, I was encouraged to leave my job. The ignorance and discrimination I have experienced has been extraordinary.'
- 'Unlike physical disability, a mental health diagnosis makes you a leper. I have had positive support in one post but been too frightened to reveal my diagnosis elsewhere. As a caring profession, medicine is very cruel to doctors with mental health problems.'
- 'After disability was disclosed through occupational health, no support was offered by trust. Instead, public humiliation increased about how I was a liability … Instead of helping, I was intentionally put in situations where I could not physically cope.'
- 'It was helpful to have some support for adjustments, however, it is then down to the practice to actually order equipment/make changes. It took the Practice Manager seven months to order the equipment funded fully by Access to Work and they refused to make the other adjustments they recommended.'

Table 8.2 Six core competencies for disability curricula recommended by the Alliance for Disability in Health Care Education (US).

Title	Competency that learners should achieve
Contextual and Conceptual Frameworks on Disability	Acquire a conceptual framework for disability in the context of human diversity, the lifespan, wellness, injury and social and cultural environments
Professionalism and Patient-Centred Care	Demonstrate mastery of general principles of professionalism, communication, respect for patients, and recognise optimal health and quality of life from the patient's perspective
Legal Obligations and Responsibilities for Caring for Patients with Disabilities	Understand and identify legal requirements for providing healthcare in a manner that is consistent with relevant national laws to meet the individual needs of people with disabilities
Teams and Systems-based Practice	Engage and collaborate with interprofessional team members within and outside their own discipline to provide high-quality, team-based healthcare to people with disabilities
Clinical Assessment	Collect and interpret relevant information about the health and function of patients with disabilities and engage patients in creating a plan of care that includes essential and optimal services and supports
Clinical Care over the Lifespan and During Transitions	Demonstrate knowledge of effective strategies to engage patients with disabilities in creating a co-ordinated plan of care with needed services and supports

Source: Adapted from Havercamp et al. [20].

Conclusion

Many factors contribute to health and healthcare disparities experienced by people with disability. Addressing these inequities will require public commitment and resources across societal sectors. Healthcare professionals should play central roles in these efforts. One starting point is undergraduate, postgraduate and continuing education programmes, which should train all healthcare professionals in basic competencies relating to disabled patients (Table 8.2).

Since many health conditions have long-term functional implications, introducing disability topics within case-based training should proceed seamlessly (e.g. case studies concerning heart failure or severe emphysema could include discussions of effects on ADLs). Such case-based teaching and other clinical training must go beyond medical model thinking to address social model and human rights concerns [20]. As Article 8, Awareness Raising, of the United Nations CRPD asserts, nations and societies need to 'combat stereotypes, prejudices and harmful practices relating to persons with disabilities … in all areas of life' and to '[foster] at all levels of the education system … an attitude of respect for the rights of persons with disabilities' [21].

Further reading/resources

Altchuler, S. (2009) Granting medical licensure, honoring the Americans with Disabilities Act, and protecting the public: can we do all three? *Academic Medicine*, **84** (6), 689–691.

Centers for Disease Control and Prevention, Disability and Health Data System (2022) 2019. Disability status and types among adults 18 years of age and older. View by: overall. Response: any disability. https://dhds.cdc.gov/LP?Ca tegoryId=DISEST&IndicatorId=STATTYPE&ShowFootnotes=true&View= Map&yearId=YR4&stratCatId1=CAT1&stratId1=BO1&stratCatId2=&strat Id2=&responseId=Q6DIS1&dataValueTypeId=AGEADJPREV&MapClassi fierId=quantile&MapClassifierCount=5 (accessed 23 April 2022)

Chen, L.S., Chou, Y.J., Tsay, J.H. et al. (2009) Variation in the cervical cancer screening compliance among women with disability. *Journal of Medical Screening*, **16** (2), 85–90.

Cohen, R.A., Gabriel, B., and Terrell, C. (2002) The case for diversity in the health care workforce. *Health Affairs*, **21** (5), 90–102.

Fragala, G. (2016) Reducing occupational risk to ambulatory caregivers. *Workplace Health and Safety*, **64** (9), 414–419.

Iezzoni, L.I., Ngo, L.H., Li, D. et al. (2008) Early-stage breast cancer treatments for younger Medicare beneficiaries with different disabilities. *Health Service Research*, **43** (5 Pt 1), 1752–1767.

Iezzoni, L.I., O'Day, B.L., Killeen, M. and Harker, H. (2004) Communicating about health care: observations from persons who are deaf or hard of hearing. *Annals of Internal Medicine*, **140** (5), 356–362.

McCarthy, E.P., Ngo, L.H., Roetzheim, R.G. et al. (2006) Disparities in breast cancer treatment and survival for women with disabilities. *Annals of Internal Medicine*, **145** (9), 637–645.

McCarthy, E.P., Ngo, L.H., Chirikos, T. et al. (2007) Cancer stage at diagnosis and survival among persons with Social Security Disability Insurance on Medicare. *Health Service Research*, **42** (2), 611–628.

Melnick, D. (2011) Balancing responsibility to patients and responsibility to aspiring physicians with disabilities. *Academic Medicine*, **86** (8), 674–676.

Olkin, R. (1999) *What Psychotherapists Should Know About Disability*. New York: Guilford Press.

Shen, M.J., Peterson, E.B., Costas-Muñiz, R. et al. (2018) The effects of race and racial concordance on patient-physician communication: a systematic review of the literature. *Journal of Racial and Ethnic Health Disparities*, **5** (1), 117–140.

Stone, D. (1984) *The Disabled State*. Philadelphia: Temple University Press.

Takeshita, J., Wang, S., Loren, A.W. and Mitra, N. (2020) Association of racial/ ethnic and gender concordance between patients and physicians with patient experience ratings. *JAMA Network Open*, **3** (11), e2024583.

World Health Organization (2001) *International Classification of Functioning, Disability and Health*. Geneva: World Health Organization.

References

1 World Health Organization and World Bank (2011) *World Report on Disability*. Geneva: WHO Press.

2 Kuper, H. and Heydt, H. (2019) The missing billion: access to health services for people with disabilities. https://www.themissingbillion.org/ the-report-2, (accessed 31 March 2022)

3 Andrews, E.E., Forber-Pratt, A.J., Mona, L.R. et al. (2019) #SaytheWord: a disability culture commentary on the erasure of 'disability'. *Rehabilitation Psychology*, **64** (2), 111–118.

4 British Medical Association (2020) Disability in the medical profession. Survey findings 2020. www.bma.org.uk/advice-and-support/equality-and-diversity-guidance/disability-equality-in-medicine/disability-in-the-medical-profession (accessed 22 April 2022)

5 Iezzoni, L.I., Rao, S.R., Agaronnik, N.D. and El-Jawahri, A. (2021a) Associations between disability and breast or cervical cancers, accounting for screening disparities. *Medical Care*, **59** (2), 139–147.

6 Marlow, N.M., Samuels, S.K. and Mainous III, A.G. (2019) Patient–provider communication quality for persons with disabilities: a cross-sectional analysis of the health information national trends survey. *Disability and Health Journal*, **12** (4), 732–737.

7 James, T.G., Coady, K.A., Stacciarini, J.-M.R. et al. (2022) 'They're not willing to accommodate deaf patients': communication experiences of deaf American sign language users in the emergency department. *Qualitative Health Research*, **32** (1), 48–63.

8 Shefer, G., Henderson, C., Howard, L.M. et al. (2014) Diagnostic overshadowing and other challenges involved in the diagnostic process of patients with mental illness who present in emergency departments with physical symptoms – a qualitative study. *PLoS One*, **9** (11), e111682.

9 Agaronnik, N.D., El-Jawahri, A. and Iezzoni, L.I. (2021) Perspectives of patients with pre-existing mobility disability on the process of diagnosing their cancer. *Journal of General Internal Medicine*, **36** (5), 1250–1257.

10 Iezzoni, L.I. (2022) Cancer detection, diagnosis, and treatment for adults with disabilities. *Lancet Oncology*, **23** (4), E164–E173.

11 Iezzoni, L.I., Rao, S.R., Ressalam, J. et al. (2021) Physicians' perceptions of people with disability and their health care. *Health Affairs*, **40** (2), 297–306.

12 Morris, M.A., Maragh-Bass, A.C., Griffin, J.M. et al. (2017) Use of accessible examination tables in the primary care setting: a survey of physical evaluations and patient attitudes. *Journal of General Internal Medicine*, **32** (12), 1342–1348.

13 Pharr, J.R., James, T. and Yeung, Y.-L. (2019) Accessibility and accommodations for patients with mobility disabilities in a large healthcare system: how are we doing? *Disability and Health Journal*, **12** (4), 679–684.

14 Iezzoni, L.I., Rao, S.R., Ressalam, J. et al. (2021c) Use of accessible weight scales and examination tables/chairs for patients with significant mobility limitations by physicians nationwide. *Joint Commission Journal on Quality and Patient Safety*, **47** (10), 615–627.

15 Iezzoni, L.I., Rao, S.R., Ressalam, J. et al. (2022) US physicians' knowledge about the Americans with Disabilities Act and accommodating patients with disability. *Health Affairs*, **41** (1), 96–104.

16 Nouri, Z., Dill, M.J., Conrad, S.S. et al. (2021) Estimated prevalence of US physicians with disabilities. *JAMA Network Open*, **4** (3), e211254.

17 Iezzoni, L.I. (2016) Why increasing numbers of physicians with disability could improve care for patients with disability. *AMA Journal of Ethics*, **18** (10), 1041–1049.

18 Meeks, L.M. and Jain, N.R. (2018) *Accessibility, Inclusion, and Action in Medical Education. Lived Experiences of Learners and Physicians with Disabilities*. Washington, DC: American Association of Medical Colleges.

19 General Medical Council (2019) Welcomed and valued: supporting disabled learners in medical education and training. www.gmc-uk.org/education/standards-guidance-and-curricula/guidance/welcomed-and-valued (accessed 22 April 2022)

20 Havercamp, S.M., Barnhart, W.R., Robinson, A.C. et al. (2021) What should we teach about disability? National consensus on disability competencies for health care education. *Disability and Health Journal*, **14** (2), 100989.

21 United Nations Department of Economic and Social Affairs (2006) Convention on the Rights of Persons with Disabilities. www.un.org/development/desa/disabilities/convention-on-the-rights-of-persons-with-disabilities/guiding-principles-of-the-convention.html (accessed 5 April 2022)

CHAPTER 9

Migrants and Displaced People

James Smith

Honorary Research Fellow, Health in Humanitarian Crises Centre, London School of Hygiene and Tropical Medicine.
Médecins Sans Frontières/Doctors Without Borders, England

OVERVIEW

- Migration and displacement are highly politicised processes, which generate and exacerbate individual health risks and vulnerabilities.
- The categories 'migrant' and 'displaced person' are representative of highly diverse groups, and as such, there is substantial heterogeneity in health needs, health outcomes and experiences of – and barriers to – accessing healthcare services within and between such groups.
- Healthcare professionals can act to improve access to and experience of healthcare services for migrants and displaced people by first recognising that systems and processes intentionally and unintentionally restrict access to healthcare for certain groups.
- A 'politicised determinants of health' approach that engages with context-specific political, economic, social and other factors that interact to affect care-seeking and health outcomes among those marginalised by society is critical to inclusive and equitable health service delivery.
- Healthcare professionals can advance inclusive and equitable service delivery by demonstrating professional curiosity regarding barriers to care and the specific experiences and needs of people accessing health services. This requires a holistic approach to health assessments ensuring that attention is paid to intersecting social issues.
- Recognition of the negative systemic impact of policies and practices on individual and population health requires that healthcare professionals participate in remedial action to counteract and ultimately dismantle the systemic causes of marginalisation and poor health.

Introduction

Ensuring health systems are responsive to the diverse needs and perspectives of migrants and displaced people is central to an inclusive and equitable healthcare system and a precondition of universal health coverage. Migrants and displaced people often face challenges accessing healthcare services (Box 9.1), and in certain situations may experience worse health outcomes compared to the general population.

Box 9.1 Challenges accessing healthcare services.

Amir was displaced by the ongoing conflict in Afghanistan and arrived in the UK after a perilous journey made necessary due to the absence of safe routes to seek protection. He speaks Pashto and very little English, and with the exception of some support from a nearby community group, has not received substantial additional assistance.

Amir has not been given information about how to navigate the UK healthcare system and cannot find information translated into Pashto. When he rings the GP surgery, the automated system does not include other languages. He waits on the line and eventually reaches a receptionist but is not provided with a translator. They repeat information in English and eventually hang up the phone. He tries unsuccessfully to make an appointment on many occasions. Eventually, another receptionist takes the time to organise a conversation using the GP practice's telephone translation service. She is able to assist Amir in registering with the practice, makes a note of his main concerns and books an appointment with the GP, while flagging that an interpreter is required and that a longer appointment slot is needed to facilitate a more detailed new patient assessment using the interpreter.

Migrants and displaced people represent vastly different groups of people, with substantial variation within and between the groups of people classified using these terms. Variation is often seen in relation to age, disability and racialised and gendered characteristics. Additionally, there is variation in the treatment of people on the move based on their country of origin and the proximity of their movement to high-income countries. As such, this chapter presents some overarching reflections intended to inform the pursuit of health equity for migrants and displaced people while avoiding overly standardised frameworks or prescriptive approaches that fail to recognise the centrality of context-specific and individualised care giving.

This chapter provides an overview of key data related to migration and displacement globally, including relevant definitions for different categorisations of people based on their migration or displacement status (Box 9.2). A short overview of predominant responses to migration and displacement is outlined before a brief analysis of risk

ABC of Equality, Diversity and Inclusion in Healthcare, First Edition. Edited by Shehla Imtiaz-Umer and John Frain.
© 2023 John Wiley & Sons Ltd. Published 2023 by John Wiley & Sons Ltd.

and vulnerability in the context of migration and displacement. This is particularly important to inform our understanding of the health needs, health outcomes, barriers to healthcare affecting people who move, and the approaches required of health professionals to ensure inclusive and equitable caregiving.

Box 9.2 Key definitions.

Migrant: a person who moves away from their place of usual residence, whether within a country or across an international border, temporarily or permanently, and for a variety of reasons.

Refugee: a person who, owing to a well-founded fear of persecution for reasons of race, religion, nationality, membership of a particular social group or political opinion, is outside the country of his nationality and is unable or, owing to such fear, is unwilling to avail himself of the protection of that country; or who, not having a nationality and being outside the country of his former habitual residence as a result of such events, is unable or, owing to such fear, is unwilling to return to it.

Asylum seeker: an individual who is seeking international protection. In countries with individualised procedures, an asylum seeker is someone whose claim has not yet been finally decided on by the country in which they submitted it.

Internally displaced person: persons or groups of persons who have been forced or obliged to flee or to leave their homes or places of habitual residence, in particular as a result of or in order to avoid the effects of armed conflict, situations of generalised violence, violations of human rights or natural or human-made disasters, and who have not crossed an internationally recognised State border.

Undocumented migrant: a non-national who enters or stays in a country without the appropriate documentation. Similar to 'Migrant in an Irregular Situation', defined as a person who moves or has moved across an international border and is not authorised to enter or to stay in a State pursuant to the law of that State and to international agreements to which that State is a party.

Source: IOM (2019) *Glossary on Migration*. Geneva: International Organisation for Migration.

Migration and displacement globally

The International Organisation for Migration (IOM) estimates that in 2020 at least 281 million people were living outside their country of origin, of which at least 169 million people were recognised as labour migrants [1]. Drivers of migration – defined as the movement of a person away from their place of usual residence [2] – are complex and often multifaceted; research has identified several dimensions spanning demographic, economic, environmental, human development, individual (e.g. resources, experiences, aspirations), politico-institutional (e.g. infrastructure, governance, policies and rights), security, sociocultural and supranational (e.g. related to globalisation, (post) colonialism, geopolitical relations) factors [3].

While many people move by choice, a growing number of people are forced to leave their homes or countries of origin. At least 96.1 million people were forcibly displaced worldwide at the end of 2021; this figure includes 59.1 million internally displaced people (IDPs) [4], 27.1 million refugees, 4.6 million asylum seekers, 4.4 million

Venezuelans displaced abroad, and 1.3 million stateless people who have been displaced, of whom the majority are Rohingya from Myanmar [5]. The majority of people forcibly displaced across a border are hosted in countries neighbouring their countries of origin. At the same time, 74% of refugees are estimated to be living in situations of protracted displacement (i.e. where 25 000 or more people are living in exile for at least five consecutive years).

An overview of global responses to migration and displacement

To better understand how to support and provide care for migrants and displaced people, it is important to be aware of some overarching trends that affect the social, political and economic conditions of people who move.

While the movement of people from one place to another has featured throughout human history, responses to migration have varied over time. They are inextricably connected to prevailing geopolitical relations and practices, notable among which are the protracted histories and contemporary manifestations of imperialism and colonialism, and broader trajectories of globalisation.

Political responses to migration have become increasingly contingent in recent decades; governments are overtly selective in the concern they display towards displaced people, and in the creation of systems that narrowly encourage only certain types of migration. This selectivity can often be distinguished based on nationality, racialised and gendered characteristics, age and presumed economic potential, among other factors. A notable recent example concerns the British government's establishment of comprehensive systems to host and support predominantly White Ukrainian refugees in early 2022 while concurrently devising plans to deport Sudanese, Iranian, Syrian and other asylum seekers to Rwanda under a scheme of questionable legality and in contravention of several human rights [6].

Relatedly, the movement of people is increasingly framed as a matter of 'high politics', i.e. concerning the state's survival, which in turn allows for migration and displacement to be presented as a threat to state security. This has been particularly apparent in the way that the movement of people into Europe since 2015 has been framed as a refugee/migration 'crisis', supposedly necessitating new and more dramatic forms of migration containment and control.

What is notable about this framing is a much greater focus by states on measures to limit the potential for movement. In some contexts, this has manifested as the externalisation of border controls, as is evident in investments made by the European Union (EU) to hinder the movement of people attempting to reach Europe from the Middle East or North Africa, such as in the case of the EU–Turkey deal [7]. Elsewhere, humanitarian and human rights monitoring organisations have witnessed pushbacks, which force the return of people to places of departure irrespective of the risk of detention, violence or persecution on their return [8]. For asylum seekers who can reach their intended destination, bureaucratic and other impediments to attaining protection result in prolonged and fraught asylum processes, which often fail to recognise the extent of an individual's protection needs. Together, these measures represent a progressive erosion of existing frameworks for legal protection.

At the same time, people who move – be it across borders or from one distinct region to another – are frequently instrumentalised for political gain. This first requires a process of 'othering' [9], which 'serves to mark and name those thought to be different from oneself' [10]. This allows for, and emboldens existing forms of, marginalisation and exclusion. A persistent consequence of such othering is the scapegoating of migrants and other marginalised groups, which allows governments to temporarily distract from the political causes of underlying social and economic problems.

Risk and vulnerability in relation to migration and displacement

For health professionals, it is particularly important to recognise that while processes of migration and displacement can present new risks to health and exacerbate pre-existing health problems (Box 9.3), it is the politicised response to the movement of people that most markedly exacerbates individual and population risk and vulnerability. Concerning migrants, the Office of the High Commissioner for Human Rights has clearly expressed that migrants 'are not inherently vulnerable, nor do they lack resilience and agency' [11]. Similarly, scholars and practitioners have increasingly challenged the complex ways in which asylum seekers, and refugees in particular, are framed as vulnerable (and therefore 'deserving' of protection) in heavily gendered and racialised ways. This is often apparent in media representations that present refugee children and women as 'deserving' and vulnerable, and refugee men as 'undeserving' and a threat [12].

Box 9.3 **Migration and displacement generating new risks to health and exacerbating existing problems.**

Kalyna and her three-year-old daughter Liliya were displaced by the Russian invasion of Ukraine. They fled overland and eventually reached Germany. Through the EU solidarity mechanism, they have been matched with a family in the UK that has offered to host the pair.

While the conflict has been traumatising, Kalyna and Liliya had to stay in four different places before reaching Germany. They were hopeful that the relocation to the UK would bring some stability. However, long delays with the visa process have left them confused and uncertain about the immediate future. Liliya is becoming increasingly unsettled and distressed.

This experience is an example of situational vulnerability.

While vulnerabilities can result from age, gender, race and other characteristics, broad claims of vulnerability can have the effect of reducing individuals to passive victims who seemingly lack agency, which in turn can be politically manipulated to present such individuals as 'needy, helpless and a drain on resources' [9].

Aside from the ways in which vulnerability can be attributed in problematic ways, it is important to discern the nuanced forms of vulnerability that may exist when providing healthcare and other essential services. Existing taxonomies have identified distinct forms of vulnerability [13], which can be broadly distinguished as follows.

- **Inherent vulnerability** – related to intrinsic characteristics connected to bodily state, dependence on others and an individual's affective and social nature.

- **Situational vulnerability** – related to the external context and influenced by personal, social, political, economic and environmental circumstances.

Both inherent and situational vulnerabilities may, in turn, be either *dispositional* (i.e. potential) or *occurrent* (i.e. actual) (Box 9.4). A further categorisation has since been proposed, which concerns 'pathogenic' vulnerability generated from responses to existing vulnerabilities that exacerbate – or generate new forms of – vulnerability [14]. This is particularly pertinent when we consider the negative consequences of state responses to migration and migrants and the negative and often traumatising effects of processes put in place to determine the protection needs and asylum claims of people seeking refuge.

Box 9.4 **From dispositional to occurrent vulnerability.**

Magdalena's parents migrated from Poland three years ago when she was 10 years old. Magdalena was born with severe physical and learning disabilities from birth and requires additional social and educational support. This is an example of an inherent vulnerability.

The family initially felt supported, their housing was appropriately adapted, Magdalena's health problems were addressed, and they felt settled within their local community. With Magdalena's additional needs, it may make her vulnerable, but in this case, she and the family have received the additional support they require, and as such the potential impact of this vulnerability has been minimised.

Due to Magdalena's mother's work, they move to a new area. After three months the parents speak to their new GP to inform them that Magdalena has still not been given a school place, their house is unsafe and damp, and the paediatric cardiology and neurology appointments she was referred for have not materialised.

This change in the family's circumstances demonstrates how the family's wider environment interacted with Magdelena's individual characteristics to generate occurrent vulnerability.

With this in mind, health professionals must develop a nuanced appreciation of how individual experiences of migration or displacement are generative of contextual and contingent forms of risk and vulnerability, which may, in turn, be intentionally or inadvertently exacerbated by measures ostensibly put in place to respond to such vulnerability.

Health needs and outcomes

As we have outlined, categories such as migrant, refugee and asylum seeker represent heterogeneous groups with distinct needs, life experiences and challenges related to access to healthcare and other essential services. An individual's environment heavily influences these needs, and conditions during a journey and after arrival (Figure 9.1). Notably, the stage and duration of migration are important factors; the health needs of newly arrived migrants and displaced people may differ substantially from the health needs of individuals who have been resettled for many years in a particular location or encamped in a single location for a prolonged period. Therefore, health professionals must be attuned to the specific challenges individuals face based on their unique experiences of migration or displacement.

That said, a comprehensive global overview of evidence compiled by the WHO in 2022 has identified patterns and trends in health

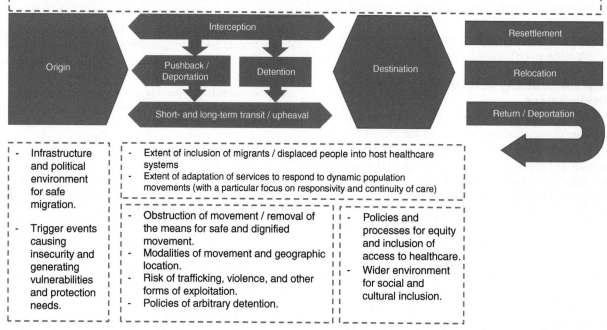

Figure 9.1 Key health-related considerations throughout processes of migration and displacement.

needs and outcomes for migrants and refugees (excluding IDPs) compared to the host population across multiple contexts, which therefore warrant brief elaboration [15]. These differences include some evidence of higher rates of occupational health-related injuries and illnesses linked to more precarious working conditions; higher rates of anaemia and malnutrition; a higher prevalence of diabetes mellitus and hypertension, which may be left uncontrolled or undiagnosed; later-stage diagnoses of cancer; higher rates of depression, anxiety and psychotic disorders, often linked to the cumulative impact of social disadvantage; higher rates of multidrug-resistant tuberculosis (MDR-TB), latent TB infection and hepatitis; and an increased risk of COVID-19 infection and severe COVID-19-related disease.

Notably, some evidence also suggests a lower awareness of available health services and utilisation of such services, particularly in relation to maternal and child health and sexual and reproductive health [15]. Additional reviews have identified lower immunisation rates among certain groups of migrants and refugees due to lower vaccination coverage rates in countries of origin [16].

It is important to stress that these are not generalisable findings. High levels of variation exist between groups and contexts, and the quality and availability of supporting evidence remain limited. This requires that contextually specific data inform health services. It is also important to recognise that data can often be skewed towards the types of health problems most often scrutinised by recipient governments and healthcare providers. As such, there is a substantial body of data related to the infectious disease profile of people on the move, which has repeatedly been used to incorrectly claim that

refugees and migrants are vectors of disease. This, in turn, has provided a 'scientific alibi' for discrimination and the contravention of human rights [17].

Recognising and addressing barriers to healthcare

As has been outlined, migrants and displaced persons are often subject to intentional forms of marginalisation and exclusion. This can be further compounded by systems and processes that are not structured to operate with a focus on inclusion and equity.

Barriers to access to healthcare may be non-specific, i.e. not targeted specifically at migrants or displaced people, such as the closure of a clinic service due to underfunding or difficulties accessing a GP due to understaffing, which affect entire communities. However, many barriers to access are targeted, whereby political decisions generate policies and practices intended to limit access to care for certain groups. This is particularly pronounced in the UK context in relation to the government's 'hostile environment' agenda. Barriers to access include individual (typically concerning factors affecting health-seeking behaviour), community, institutional and structural factors (Figure 9.2) These factors can interact positively and negatively to shape access to healthcare. For example, access barriers at the individual level (such as a fear of seeking care) often result from – or are amplified by – structural and other factors (such as government policies that require health facilities to share patient information with immigration services).

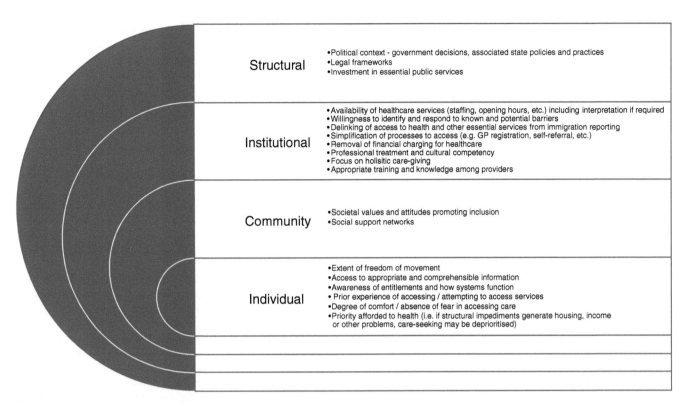

Figure 9.2 Barriers to accessing healthcare.

The role of health professionals working with migrants and displaced people

As emphasised elsewhere in this book, healthcare provider responsibilities extend beyond the clinical elements of an individual patient encounter. This may be more immediately apparent for professional cadres who engage with patients over a prolonged time in the community setting and who more frequently encounter how our social, economic and political environment impacts health. However, this responsibility extends as much to general surgeons, hospital physiotherapists and paediatric emergency nurses as it does to general practitioners, community social workers and housing officers.

This can be achieved by taking time to build relationships with patients, displaying professional curiosity and ensuring sensitive enquiry when seeking to understand individual life stories and experiences (Box 9.5). This is particularly important given that a lack of trust in the healthcare system and fear of healthcare providers are frequently cited as barriers to accessing healthcare among migrants and marginalised groups.

Box 9.5 Professional curiosity and building relationships.

Jemal fled Eritrea 18 months ago. He travelled through Sudan and Libya where he was caught and detained in a squalid detention facility. Eventually, he was able to travel by boat and was rescued by an NGO vessel. Those rescued were held at sea for 10 days before Italy assigned a safe port.

Jemal travelled through Europe and was stuck in the makeshift camps in Calais for many months. There, he was beaten and tear-gased on two separate occasions by the notorious French CRS police service. He eventually reached the UK and was able to make an asylum claim.

He has since registered with a GP and has attended several times in the last two months with a variety of complaints: first a persistent headache, then difficulty sleeping, and now generalised aches and abdominal pain. Jemal is seen by a number of different GPs but is eventually seen by a GP who saw him during one of his earlier appointments. Jemal makes a passing reference to his asylum claim, and the GP asks if he feels comfortable speaking about his experience. Jemal proceeds to describe not only what happened in Eritrea, but the prolonged and traumatic experience he endured in order to reach the UK. Having ruled out possible physical causes for these complaints, the GP is concerned these changing symptoms may be more somatic in nature. This is broached with Jemal who divulges feeling low in mood and increasingly anxious. He agrees to a referral for mental health input, while the GP arranges a follow-up appointment for the following week, making a note that Jemal should preferably be seen by the same GP if possible. In the meantime, the GP also arranges to speak to an advisory service that specialises in providing support to people who have experienced detention.

Furthermore, in recognition of the systemic policies and practices that negatively affect access to and the availability of healthcare services for migrants, displaced people and other marginalised groups, it is important that healthcare professionals and allied colleagues proactively advocate for healthcare systems that emulate the principles of inclusion and equity, while simultaneously obstructing and exposing policies and practices that undermine those principles.

Further reading/resources

Asif, Z. and Kienzler, H. (2022) Structural barriers to refugee, asylum seeker and undocumented migrant healthcare access. Perceptions of Doctors of the World caseworkers in the UK. *SSM – Mental Health*, **2**, 100088.

Bivins, R. (2015) *Contagious Communities: Medicine, Migration, and the NHS in Post-War Britain*. Oxford: Oxford University Press.

BMA (2019) *BMA Refugee and Asylum Seeker Health Resource*. London: British Medical Association.

Lessard-Phillips, L. et al. (2021) *Barriers to Wellbeing. Migration and Vulnerability During the Pandemic*. London: Doctors of the World UK.

Matlin, S.A. et al. (2018) Migrants' and refugees' health: towards an agenda of solutions. *Public Health Reviews*, **39**: 27.

OHCHR (n.d.) Principles and guidelines on the human rights protection of migrants in vulnerable situations. www.ohchr.org/sites/default/files/Documents/Issues/Migration/PrinciplesAndGuidelines.pdf (accessed 8 October 2022)

Spitzer, D.L. et al. (2019) Towards inclusive migrant healthcare. *BMJ*, **366**, I4256.

Tomkow, L.J. et al. (2020) Healthcare access for asylum seekers and refugees in England: a mixed methods study exploring service users' and health care professionals' awareness. *European Journal of Public Health*, **30** (3), 527–532.

Worthing, K. et al. (2021) Patients or passports? The 'hostile environment' in the NHS. *Future Healthcare Journal*, **8** (1), 28–30.

References

1 IOM (2021) *World Migration Report 2022*. Geneva: International Organisation for Migration.

2 IOM (2019) *Glossary on Migration*. Geneva: International Organisation for Migration.

3 Czaika, M. and Reinprecht, C. (2020) *Drivers of Migration: A Synthesis of Knowledge*. Amsterdam: International Migration Institute.

4 IDMC (2022) *Global Report on Internal Displacement 2022*. Geneva: Internal Displacement Monitoring Centre.

5 UNHCR (2022) *Global Trends Forced Displacement in 2021*. Geneva: United Nations High Commissioner for Refugees.

6 Balogun-Mwangi, O. (2022) Disparities in global empathy: why some refugees are more welcome than others. https://theconversation.com/disparities-in-global-empathy-why-some-refugees-are-more-welcome-than-others-184171 (accessed 21 September 2022)

7 Mussa, R. (2021) Fifth anniversary of the EU-Turkey deal: EU leaders celebrate years of chaos and mistreatment. https://msf-analysis.org/fifth-anniversary-of-the-eu-turkey-deal-eu-leaders-celebrate-years-of-chaos-and-mistreatment (accessed 25 September 2022).

8 Tondo, L. (2021) Revealed: 2,000 refugee deaths linked to illegal EU pushbacks. https://www.theguardian.com/global-development/2021/may/05/revealed-2000-refugee-deaths-linked-to-eu-pushbacks (accessed 25 September 2022)

9 Grove N.J. and Zwi, A. (2006) Our health and theirs: forced migration, othering, and public health. *Scoial Science and Medicine*, **62**, 1931–1942.

10 Weis, L. (1995) Identity formation and the process of 'othering': unravelling sexual threads. *Journal of Educational Foundations*, **9** (1), 17–33.

11 OHCHR (2018) Principles and guidelines, supported by practical guidance, on the human rights protection of migrants in vulnerable situations. Geneva: Office of the United Nations High Commissioner for Human Rights.

12 Gray, H. et al. (2019) Refugees as/at risk: the gendered and racialized underpinnings of securitization in British media narratives. *Security Dialogue*, **50** (3), 275–291.

13 Mackenzie, C. et al. (2014) Introduction: what is vulnerability and why does it matter for moral theory? In: *Vulnerability. New Essays in Ethics and Feminist Philosophy* (eds W. Rogers et al.). Oxford: Oxford University Press.

14 Rogers et al. (2012) Why bioethics needs a concept of vulnerability. *International Journal of Feminist Approaches to Bioethics*, **5** (2), 11–38.

15 WHO (2022) *World Report on the Health of Refugees and Migrants*. Geneva: World Health Organization.

16 Mipatrini, D. et al. (2017) Vaccinations in migrants and refugees: a challenge for European health systems. A systematic review of current scientific evidence. *Pathogens and Global Health*, **111** (2), 59–68.

17 Khan, M.S. et al. (2016) Pathogens, prejudice, and politics: the role of the global health community in the European refugee crisis. *Lancet Infectious Diseases*, **16** (8), E173–E177.

CHAPTER 10

Mental Health

Oluwaseun Oluwaranti

Higher Trainee in Forensic Psychiatry, Nottinghamshire Healthcare NHS Foundation Trust, Nottingham, UK

OVERVIEW

- People with marginalised identities are often treated and perceived differently by others.
- Their experience may make them vulnerable to developing mental health problems.
- Service users with protected characteristics are likely to suffer discrimination when accessing health services, including mental health.
- A multilevel approach is needed to address the difference and to improve outcomes.

Introduction

The impact of marginalised identities on a person's wellbeing is discussed elsewhere (see Chapters 6, 7 and 11). It is worth considering, in more detail, the impact of mental health conditions on patients with protected characteristics, as it can be severe. It can affect the person's ability to access services, disclose aspects of their history and identity and reduce both quality of life and long-term survival. This chapter will examine how mental health disorders intersect and interact with marginalised identities. This includes not only the impact of mental health disorders on individuals themselves but also how healthcare organisations treat them.

Mental health and protected characteristics

About one in six adults in the United Kingdom has a common mental health disorder (Box 10.1) [1]. However, not all mental health problems or disorders are considered disabilities. The Equality Act 2010 (henceforth referred to as the Act) is focused on a set of characteristics that aims to protect people with 'protected characteristics' from discrimination and other forms of unfair treatment.

Box 10.1 **Common mental disorders.**

Under the Equality Act 2010, protection can be given where a mental health condition is proven to be a disability as defined under the Act. Criteria demonstrating disability include the following.
- The condition has more than a small impact on the patient's everyday life.
- It makes life more difficult for the patient.
- It has lasted at least 12 months, is likely to last 12 months or if improvement has occurred, it is likely to recur.
Examples of mental health conditions which may qualify as disabilities include:
- anxiety
- bipolar disorder
- body dysmorphic disorder
- borderline personality disorder
- depression
- eating problems
- obsessive-compulsive disorders
- posttraumatic stress disorder
- schizophrenia.
People may have mental health conditions which do not reach the threshold of disability but nonetheless affect the impact of other protected characteristics.

Source: MIND: www.mind.org.uk

While the Act does not directly cover mental health, it provides broader coverage for disabilities arising from any cause, including mental health conditions. A mental health condition becomes a disability when it has a lasting impact on one's ability to perform normal daily activities such as caring for oneself and others, communication and movement.

People with mental health problems, especially severe mental illness, face exclusion and discrimination on many levels. Some may be as a direct result of the mental illness and its impact on the person; others

---

ABC of Equality, Diversity and Inclusion in Healthcare, First Edition. Edited by Shehla Imtiaz-Umer and John Frain.
© 2023 John Wiley & Sons Ltd. Published 2023 by John Wiley & Sons Ltd.

are related to structural, systemic and societal responses to people with mental health conditions [2].

Before the era of humane treatment and the recognition of the biological basis of mental health conditions, people with mental disorders were subjected to treatment meant for slaves and criminals (which in current-day parlance of those words would fail to convey the horrors of such treatment) such as torture, banishment, chaining, burning or killing.

There is robust research into how differently people with mental health conditions or any characteristics that are not the 'norm' are treated or perceived by others and sometimes by themselves. The early work of Erving Goffman on stigma [3], and other more recent studies, recognised that stigma and discrimination against people with mental illness are important correlates of help-seeking behaviour, recovery, integration back into society, relapse and suicide [4,5].

There are also theories on the aetiological roles of social adversities and environmental stressors in the development of mental health problems. It is widely acknowledged that these relationships are complex and potentially bidirectional (Figure 10.1) [6].

Social causation of mental disorders

The cause of mental disorders is complex and multifactorial; it is viewed as being the interaction of biological, psychological and social factors.

The social causation theory of mental disorders focuses largely on socioeconomic deprivation and mental illness and has inequality, discrimination and poor representation of people in lower classes at its core [7]. Many parallels of socioeconomic deprivation can be found in people excluded or deprived for any reason.

In addition, social causation theories, in contrast to biological and sometimes psychological causal processes, attribute causation to larger societal factors or an individual's personal circumstances.

Exclusion, discrimination or lack of representation place significant stress on the individual and limit their ability to cope resourcefully with such stressors. People with protected characteristics may, in addition to their characteristics, have mental health problems which may be exacerbated by their protected attributes, unlike those without such attributes.

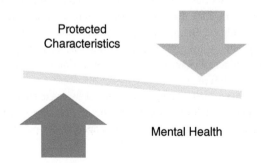

Figure 10.1 Bidirectional relationship between mental health and protected characteristics. The experience of discrimination, exclusion and inequity among people with protected characteristics makes them vulnerable to developing mental health problems.

Mental health problems (as a general condition, not considering peculiarities of specific disorders) cut across all strata of society however we choose to consider it; they can affect all age groups, social classes, sexual orientations, races, etc.

The approach to prevention, service provision, care and management should be tailored in such a way that this distribution is reflected; however, those with characteristics outside the 'norm' may be easily excluded from such interventions.

Impact of protected characteristics on mental health

Protected characteristics are factors pertaining to us all in one way or another; we primarily have an origin which is race/ethnicity and fall into a certain sex classification (or not) or age category. Other characteristics such as marriage, pregnancy, sexual orientation, religion/beliefs, disability or gender reassignment are perhaps consequences of living themselves, which are important parts of self-definition, identity and connectedness. Hence, protected characteristics may be things we have little choice about and/or are integral to who we are. The definition of mental health as:

> the state of mental wellbeing that enables people to cope with the stresses of life, realise their abilities, learn and work well, and contribute to their community [8]

shows that limitation of an individual or group based on any of the protected characteristics or other attributes is likely to affect their mental health negatively.

There is limited collective research on protected characteristics, perhaps because it covers a wide range of attributes that makes focusing on all at once cumbersome or because one characteristic may confound findings in the research of others. Although we often try to look at these attributes as singular entities, no protected characteristic exists by itself (see Chapter 11).

Mental health disparities related to race, gender, disabilities and sexual orientation are more prominent in research and will be discussed later. Others, such as age, pregnancy and marriage, are less well covered in research but certainly not of lesser significance.

Age

The world is full of opportunities that sometimes balance themselves over the course of one's life and are spread across age groups. Worldwide, there is an emphasis on the protection of people at the extremes of ages based on their vulnerabilities. We see it sometimes in railcard discounts, elderly bus passes or no payment for children under five years. Nonetheless, there are societal roles that one is expected to attain at a certain age/age group; hence, age discrimination is often subtle, somewhat tolerated and largely underresearched compared with other protected characteristics [9].

A longitudinal study of 7731 people aged 50 and older in England reported that 25.1% of participants in the study reported perceived age discrimination (Box 10.2). Perceived discrimination was associated with increased odds of poor self-rated health, depressive symptoms and chronic illnesses over six years [9].

Box 10.2 **Ageism and mental health.**

During the COVID-19 pandemic, ageist attitudes could be identified through the experience of residents in care homes, decisions on hospital admission and attitudes of younger people towards lockdown restrictions and protecting the old.

Structural ageism includes:
- denial of access to healthcare
- rationing of medical services on grounds of age
- the elderly being excluded from research and clinical trials
- reduced employment opportunities for older people.

Individuals may also internalise stereotypes about ageing throughout their lives, thus affecting their wellbeing and physical health as they age.

Source: mentalhealthandaging.com

Other studies have reported negative self-perception, poorer life satisfaction and low self-esteem because of discrimination. A review of ageism posited that negative stereotypes about ageing might overestimate the cognitive difficulties experienced by older people [10].

A spectrum of mental health problems is impacted by age, including fear of changing roles in society and organisations, loss of friends and family or staying relevant. Conversely, younger age groups suffer from a lack of confidence, identity crises, anxiety about role transitions and substance use.

Service provisions are also sometimes artificially demarcated by age boundaries with the sudden termination of care once a certain age threshold is reached. This may lead to worsening mental health conditions as the individual struggles to form a therapeutic alliance with the new team (Box 10.3).

Box 10.3 **Moving from childhood to adulthood.**

Flo was attacked over the school holidays when she was 14. She suffered from increasing anxiety and became suicidal. Thankfully she received help from the Children and Adolescent Health Services over the following four years. Her problems were found to be associated with childhood abuse by her stepfather, aged 3–5 years.

Flo needed psychotherapy and was starting to develop skills of resilience and had plans to go to college and start a course in childcare. She was suddenly told by her support worker that, due to her age, she would soon be transferred to adult services. Nobody explained what that would mean. She had really started to trust her psychologist. There was no real closure and she found herself on a waiting list which, she was told, could be up to a year.

She started to self-harm. What was the point? No-one cared about her at all. She was just a number. All the support she had received seemed really hollow and the promises had been broken.

All she needed was someone to talk to her and to follow her through the transition from child to adult services, and without that, she felt everything was falling apart.

Gender

The problems of age are amplified when viewed through the lens of gender, with women often holding the shorter end of the stick. The largely patriarchal system of most societies meant women inherited historical disadvantages which persist in some developing countries and sadly metamorphosed into different forms in its expression in modern societies. As a result, women have been pervasive victims in almost all imaginable contexts.

Women are often victims of rape and abuse in war; they are also disproportionally overrepresented in caring/caregiving in families during war and peace. At home, they may experience domestic violence, financial exploitation and poor support during pregnancy.

In the workplace, they are often subjected to harassment and have to put their careers on hold when pregnant. In some developing countries, a premium is placed on having male children while females are excluded from schools and learning. In developed countries, there is underpayment and underrepresentation in leadership positions.

These experiences create vulnerabilities that predispose women to mental health problems. Females have about twice the risk of depression and anxiety compared to males; they also have a higher risk of self-harm and posttraumatic stress disorder (PTSD) (Box 10.4).

Box 10.4 **Effects of a history of abuse.**

Maisie, a 24-year-old single mum, came to see her GP. She was struggling to cope with her two young children. Maisie explained that she had been in an abusive relationship which echoed her childhood living with an alcoholic and abusive father. Maisie was afraid that social services would take her children away, so she had not come for help. She had started to self-harm by cutting her thighs and wrists. It relieved the stress for a short while, but the emotional pain kept returning. Eventually, her friend, noticing the cuts on the wrists, persuaded Maisie to seek help. Maisie could not sleep, her appetite was poor and she had become increasingly anxious. She denied any suicidal ideas or plans but continued to contemplate self-harm.

Maisie was signposted to cognitive behaviour therapy (CBT) services, women's support groups and regular reviews with the GP.

Victims of childhood and domestic abuse are at higher risk of mood disorders and anxiety; rape victims may have PTSD and other psychological problems, affecting their ability to form mutually beneficial relationships with others. Poor progress with a career and a sense of disenfranchisement affect self-esteem and limit productivity.

Males are also often viewed as 'macho' and could be at the receiving end in abusive relationships or as a victim of parental abuse in childhood. They are more likely to be victims of violent crimes and are often raised with stereotypes and biases that are unhelpful to their mental health. This may manifest as a problem with help seeking when unwell and inappropriate coping mechanisms leading them to maladaptively use substances or commit suicide. Males are more likely to be homeless, imprisoned or die by suicide (Box 10.5).

Box 10.5 **Homophobic assault and suicidal plans.**

Paul and Jason had been together for two years. Jason had been struggling with low mood since a serious homophobic assault six months ago. He had become isolated from his Nigerian family, who rejected his relationship. They were both working, but Jason had been worried about making mistakes due to poor concentration. Paul was supportive but could not seem to help. Jason could not sleep, lost weight and became more withdrawn. He struggled to leave the house due to severe anxiety, fearing another attack.

Paul persuaded him to seek help, and he visited his GP surgery. His GP listened to the history, and Paul was shocked to hear Jason admit suicidal ideas and that he had planned to kill himself by hanging. Jason had bought the rope on the internet the previous week and had been waiting until Paul was on nights the following week.

Jason was seen that day by the Crisis Team, who diagnosed post-traumatic stress disorder (PTSD) and severe depression. Jason received intense therapy and support for the next year.

For a long time, the idea of binary and static gender/gender identity was the predominant view entertained by most of society; opinions on sexual orientation were narrow and influenced largely by religious and political views. Current understanding of gender/gender identity and sexual orientation, especially in developed and liberal countries, considers it as a spectrum that is fluid and non-binary (see Chapter 7).

Individuals belonging to this group often experience stigma and discrimination. This may occur due to family rejection, self-rejection, conversion therapy, bullying in school or victimisation and poor support at work. Studies have found that this group is at higher risk of developing mental disorders such as anxiety, depression, substance use and suicide (Figure 10.2) [11].

Mental health problems experienced by minority groups

There is a robust body of research on minority groups (Box 10.6), perhaps more than the other protected characteristics; this has helped to improve our knowledge and understanding of some of the factors

that are peculiar to the group. It has also raised important discussions about the general treatment of the minority population, generated policies and influenced service provision and delivery.

Box 10.6 **Definition of a minority.**

The minority is best captured by the definition 'any small group in society that is different from the rest because of their race, religion, or political beliefs, or a person who belongs to such a group'[12].

It is important to understand that no minority is a single entity containing identical individuals but is a diverse range of people, practices and opinions. This explains why Black, Asian and minority ethnic (BAME) is an unsatisfactory term, being too simplistic and not reflective of the range of ethnicities in society.

Similarly, terms such as LGBT, LGBTQ or LGBTQIA+ include lesbian, gay, bisexual, transgender, questioning, queer, intersex, asexual, pansexual and allies. This is important in considering each community's mental health and other needs, particularly when individuals hold multiple identities.

From definition and experience, the minority comprises complex heterogeneous groups with intra- and intergroup diversity; their reported challenges are often a mesh of collective experiences that misses out on significant nuances of component groups.

In this narrative, like most others, the term 'minority' will primarily refer to the 'racial' component of the definition. (It will be used to briefly describe mental health and the protected characteristic of sexual orientation.) However, it is recognised that every race has its predominant religion(s), culture and values, which greatly influence their way of life and perception.

While the Black, minority ethnic (BME) and Black, Asian and minority ethnic (BAME) acronyms attempt to capture and represent a collective, they were recognised as divisive and discriminatory in focus. On the surface, they cover Black, Asian and Minority ethnic groups but captured within the definition are many people who do not feel they belong to the group or are defined by it. The term is no longer used in government and other institutions. However, there is ongoing use of these terms in some spheres as there is recognition of the difficulty of a suitable alternative term.

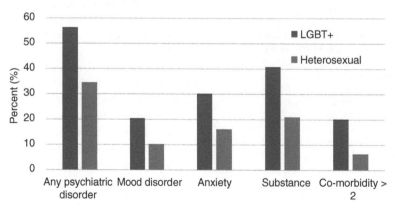

Figure 10.2 Sexual orientation disparities in psychiatric morbidity.
Source: Hatzenbuehler, M.L., Keyes, K.M., Hasin, D.S. (2009) State-level policies and psychiatric morbidity in lesbian, gay, and bisexual populations. *American Journal of Public Health* 99(1), 2275–2281.

Prevalence

Many studies have reported a higher prevalence of both common and severe mental disorders in minority groups in the UK [13,14]. These rates are higher than the prevalence rate of the disorders in their local communities. People of Black and Asian origin have higher rates of common mental disorders, with Asian females having a higher risk of anxiety and depressive disorders [13]. For psychotic disorders, the findings of higher rates of psychosis in Blacks of Caribbean and African origins have been consistent in studies (Box 10.7) [14].

Box 10.7 **Psychotic illness in a man of Afro-Caribbean descent.**

Martha was desperate. Her 21-year-old son's behaviour was becoming increasingly bizarre. Will had been close to his Uncle Max, who returned to Jamaica when he was diagnosed with terminal cancer. Martha had assumed this was the cause of Will's change in personality but on reflection, things had been deteriorating for many months. Will had been doing well at university. He was a computer whizz and seemed to be popular and happy.

When lockdown came, he seemed to adjust and continued to do his dissertation from his shared house. His friend Nick rang Martha and explained that Will just did not come out of his room. He was not eating or washing. He refused to share the chores or bills with his friends. Nick started to become afraid for his friend when Will began to pull all the plugs out and smashed the television saying that the government were communicating through the cables.

Martha tried to phone Will, but there was no answer. Nick explained that Will had destroyed his phone, fearing that he was being monitored and spied on. She went to see Will, who refused to let her into his room. He was distressed, shouting that she was being watched and monitored.

He had always been so quiet, gentle and calm. Martha knew they had to seek urgent help for Will even though he adamantly and violently refused when she suggested this to him.

Factors associated with these findings other than the stress of migration include racial discrimination, lack of inclusion and higher inequality. Some factors, such as overdiagnosis and misidentification of mental disorders, have also been suggested to explain the differences.

Individuals of minority origin are at different levels of generational, sociocultural, economic and psychological adaptation to their environment, which influences resilience and vulnerabilities to challenges of inequalities, exclusivity and monoculturalism.

Disorders such as anxiety, depression, substance use and PTSD could be explained as a direct consequence of the discrimination experienced by inequalities of the minority; psychosis and severe mood disorders are more likely due to complex and indirect results of these experiences.

Disparities in the mental health of minorities

Other studies have reported that when factors such as age, gender, race and socioeconomic differences are controlled for, there is little difference in the prevalence of mental disorders in minority groups compared to the general population [13,15]. However, evidence that mental health problems persist in minorities compared to the native population and that outcomes are poorer for minorities is unequivocal [16].

This differential mental health outcome, or disparity, can be related to any of the protected characteristics; however, it is commonly used for differences based on race, social class and sexual orientation.

A narrative review of mental health disparities of people with severe mental illness found that Blacks and ethnic minorities were more likely to receive a diagnosis of schizophrenia than the White population. Minorities also had higher doses of medication and more long-acting injections and were likely to present via emergency services [17].

A review commissioned by NHS England to examine the evidence for racial disparities in mental health in England also highlighted differences in the mental health of minorities compared to the White population from diagnosis to recovery [18].

There was evidence that Black and minority groups were less likely to access services and more likely to be referred through the criminal justice system, experienced ethnic bias and uncertainty in diagnosis, were more likely to be medicated and had poorer recovery based on their experience.

Perhaps no other disparity evidence could be more apparent than the racial and ethnic issues identified by the review of the Mental Health Act. This legislation covers the compulsory treatment of people with mental illness (Box 10.8).

Box 10.8 **Ethnic and racial differences identified in Mental Health Act (MHA) review.**

- There is variation in compulsory detention and treatment across ethnic groups.
- Most ethnic minorities in the UK are more likely to be detained than their White counterparts.
- Use of the MHA is especially high in the Black Caribbean, Black African and Black British populations.
- Disparities are driven by wider inequalities within and beyond the mental health community.
- Black or Black British people are more likely:
  - to be detained for longer
  - to experience repeated admission
  - to be subject to MHA detention power used by the police.
- There is a lack of research on detention in ethnic groups.
- MIND reported that many experience detention not as 'a therapeutic intervention, but as … chemical and physical containment.'

Source: UK Parliament Postnote 671 May 2022. Mental Health Act Reform – Race and Ethnic Inequalities. https://researchbriefings.files.parliament.uk/documents/POST-PN-0671/POST-PN-0671.pdf

---

The review identified a disproportionate number of Black and minority groups detained under the Mental Health Act. Black patients are disproportionately subjected to restrictive practices such as hospital admission, physical restraints and community treatment orders [19]. Overall, it reported profound inequalities for people from ethnic minority communities regarding access to treatment, care experiences and care outcomes. It noted that the experiences of those of Black African and Caribbean heritage are those of being either excluded or detained.

Table 10.1 Overview of strategies to reduce mental health disparities.

Factors	General initiatives	Service provider	Service user
Stigma/ discrimination	Anti-stigma campaign by popular figures and community leaders. Outreach efforts and media campaigns. Provision of non-traditional services such as home visits	Interpersonal contact between provider and patient. Cultural champions and brokers in programme development	Engagement in peer support. Engagement in specific stigma reduction psychosocial strategies
Mistrust of service	Representation and diversity in workforce. Cultural competency training	Collaborative care. Tailored interventions that are culturally and context relevant. Acknowledging failures or limitation when present	Shared decision making between carer and patient. Service user feedback and action
Family support	Family-focused interventions in community setting	Acknowledgement of family distress and offering support. Key worker to liaise with family	Working with family in treatment planning. Progress update
Culture/religion	Culturally sensitive programme development among stakeholders. Presentation and delivery of services in acceptable public settings such as churches, schools or communal meetings	Due consideration for religious and cultural values. Assessment of cultural/religious values and needs. Promote competencies in carers	Engagement in adapted cultural/ religious interventions

Source: Adapted from Maura and Weisman [17].

Sexual minorities also experience higher rates of mental disorders than the majority; they are also more likely to use mental health services and have higher rates of disability [20].

Although it is acknowledged that the factors driving disparities are complex, structural and systemic discrimination of minorities in care and service provision is often a common theme. Other factors include delayed presentation, internalised stigma, cultural beliefs about illness, mistrust and perception of service, and socioeconomic deprivation [17].

While these differences are striking, if not distressing, they have informed changes in policies and legislation. An example of this is the recently enacted Seni's law or Mental Health Units (Use of Force) Act, which is named after Olaseni Lewis, a Black male who died in 2010 following prolonged restraint by police officers while in a mental health hospital.

The inquest into his death found that the restraint used was 'disproportionate and unreasonable' and contributed to his death. The law ensures better patient protection through greater accountability and transparency in using restraints in mental health settings.

Some factors identified to combat the disparities include increased efforts at reducing stigma, culturally sensitive interventions, building trust in the system and greater involvement of families in care. These can be deployed at different intervention levels, as described in Maura and Weismann's review (Table 10.1).

Conclusion

The Equality Act has within its powers protection against discrimination based on protected characteristics as recognised under the Act. However, finer shades of support or strategies are sometimes needed to identify and enable it to discharge its powers.

There is a bidirectional relationship between protected characteristics and mental health; evidence suggests that the experiences of people with protected characteristics, such as discrimination, exclusion and inequality, make them vulnerable to developing mental health problems. Sexual and ethnic minorities experience significant disparities in terms of prevalence, health-seeking behaviour and mental health outcomes.

It is hoped that reform of the Mental Health Act would address some of these disparities; however, it is important to recognise that some of the identified differences occurred within existing legislation. Beyond laws and policies, safeguards for monitoring and compliance will be key to delivering the goals of the reform.

Further reading/resources

Mental Health Foundation. www.mentalhealth.org.uk/explore-mental-health/a-z-topics/black-asian-and-minority-ethnic-bame-communities (accessed 24 October 2022)

Rethink Mental Illness. http://www.rethink.org/get-involved/campaign-with-us/rights-involvement-and-co-production/senis-law (accessed 24 October 2022)

Writing about ethnicity. https://www.ethnicity-facts-figures.service.gov.uk/ (accessed 24 October 2022)

References

1 Mcmanus, S., Bebbington, P., Jenkins, R. et al. (2016) Mental Health and Wellbeing in England: Adult Psychiatric Morbidity Survey 2014 Executive Summary. https://assets.publishing.service.gov.uk/government/uploads/system/uploads/attachment_data/file/556596/apms-2014-full-rpt.pdf

2 Rössler, W. (2016) The stigma of mental disorders: a millennia-long history of social exclusion and prejudices. *EMBO Reports*, **17**, 9.

3 Goffman, E. (1963) *Stigma: Notes on the Management of Spoiled Identity*. London: Penguin.

4 Corrigan, P.W. and Watson, A.C. (2002) Understanding the impact of stigma on people with mental illness. *World Psychiatry*, **1** (1), 16–29.

5 Thornicroft, G. (2008) Stigma and discrimination limit access to mental health care. *Epidemiologia e Psichiatria Sociale*, **17**, 14–19.

6 Agid, O., Kohn, Y. and Lerer, B. (2000). Environmental stress, and psychiatric illness. *Biomedicine and Pharmacotherapy*, **54**, 3.

7 Peng, C.J. (2009) Sociological theories relating to mental disabilities in racial and ethnic minority populations. *Journal of Human Behavior in the Social Environment*, **19**, 85–98.

8   World Health Organization (2004)*Promoting Mental Health: Concepts, Emerging Evidence, Practice: Summary Report.* Geneva: World Health Organization.

9   Jackson, S.E., Hackett, R.A. and Steptoe, A. (2019) Associations between age discrimination and health and wellbeing: cross-sectional and prospective analysis of the English Longitudinal Study of Ageing. *Lancet Public Health*, **4** (4), e200–e208.

10 Marquet, M., Missotten, P. and Adam, S. (2019) Ageism, and overestimation of cognitive difficulties in older people: a review. *Geriatrie et Psychologie Neuropsychiatrie du Vieillisement*, **14** (2), 177–186.

11 King, M., Semlyen, J., Tai, S.S. et al. (2008) A systematic review of mental disorder, suicide, and deliberate self-harm in lesbian, gay and bisexual people. *BMC Psychiatry*, **8**, 70.

12 Cambridge University Press (2020) *Cambridge Dictionary: English Dictionary, Translations & Thesaurus.* Cambridge: Cambridge University Press.

13 Ahmad, G., McManus, S., Cooper, C. et al. (2022) Prevalence of common mental disorders and treatment receipt for people from ethnic minority backgrounds in England: repeated cross-sectional surveys of the general population in 2007 and 2014. *British Journal of Psychiatry*, **221** (3), 520–527.

14 Qassem, T., Bebbington, P., Spiers, N. et al. (2015) Prevalence of psychosis in black ethnic minorities in Britain: analysis based on three national surveys. *Social Psychiatry and Psychiatric Epidemiology*, **50** (7), 1057–1064.

15 Breslau, J., Kendler, K.S., Su, M. et al. (2005) Lifetime risk and persistence of psychiatric disorders across ethnic groups in the United States. *Psychological Medicine*, **35** (3), 317–327.

16 McGuire, T.G. and Miranda, J. (2008) Racial and ethnic disparities in mental health care: evidence and policy implications. *Health Affairs*, **27** (2), 393–403.

17 Maura, J. and Weisman de Mamani, A. (2017) Mental health disparities, treatment engagement, and attrition among racial/ethnic minorities with severe mental illness: a review. *Journal of Clinical Psychology in Medical Settings*, **24**, 187–210.

18 Bignall, T., Jeraj, S., Helsby, E. and Butt, J. (2019) Racial disparities in mental health: literature and evidence review. https://raceequalityfoundation.org.uk/wp-content/uploads/2022/10/mental-health-report-v5-2.pdf

19 Department of Health and Social Care (2018) *Modernising the Mental Health Act: Increasing Choice, Reducing Compulsion. Final Report of the Independent Review of the Mental Health Act 1983.* London: Department of Health and Social Care.

20 Cochran, S.D., Björkenstam, C. and Mays, V.M. (2017) Sexual orientation differences in functional limitations, disability, and mental health services use: results from the 2013–2014 national health interview survey. *Journal of Consulting and Clinical Psychology*, **85** (12), 1111–1121.

CHAPTER 11

Privilege, Power and Intersectionality in Healthcare

Shehla Imtiaz-Umer

Equality, Diversity and Inclusion (EDI) Director, General Practice Task Force (GPTF) Derbyshire, UK; General Practitioner, UK; GMC Associate, UK

OVERVIEW

- Privilege operates at the personal, interpersonal, cultural and institutional levels, bestowing advantages, favours and benefits on people depending on their social identity.
- The power that we hold is intricately linked to the privileges that we hold.
- Intersectionality promotes an understanding of humans as being shaped by the interaction of different social identities.
- The lack of power and privilege of some people reflects their intersectional identities and causes them to suffer oppression and prejudice.
- There needs to be increased recognition of the importance of intersectionality in interpersonal interactions but also how it can be integrated into research and policy decisions to ensure health and social equity.

Introduction

Everyone has many social identities [1] such as gender, ethnicity, race, (dis)ability, sexuality, religion or any other part of our identity. Intersectionality is defined as 'the interconnected nature of social categorisations such as race, class, and gender, regarded as creating overlapping and interdependent systems of discrimination or disadvantage'. Before considering the idea of intersectionality in the context of healthcare, it is essential to reflect on the influence of power and privilege on the identities of some people and the oppression of others.

Privilege

'Privilege exists when one group has something of value that is denied to others simply because of the groups they belong to, rather than because of anything they've done or failed to do. Access to privilege doesn't determine one's outcomes, but it is definitely an asset that makes it more likely that whatever talent, ability, and aspirations a person with privilege has will result in something positive for them.'

(Peggy McIntosh [2])

Privilege operates at the personal, interpersonal, cultural and institutional levels, bestowing advantages, favours and benefits on people depending on their social identity [1]. Put simply, it is when you think something is not a problem because it's not a problem for you personally.

Within each social identity is a hierarchy – a social status with a 'dominant group' and a 'non-dominant' group. The dominant group privilege bestows benefits to members they see as being within their 'norm' at the expense of non-dominant group members [1]. People who belong to one or more of the dominant social identity groups are given special treatment depending on the value that the specific society places on the various privileges (Figure 11.1).

Social identities, however, are always bound by their context. For example, being a consultant cardiologist will provide status and privilege within the hospital. If that consultant were on a train, that social identity would be meaningless.

Simply belonging to a dominant group allows people to move more easily through the world. They have access to resources to achieve their goals and acquire more power, thereby maintaining dominance within that social identity. The lack of privilege afforded to people from non-dominant groups makes success more difficult. They are given fewer first and second chances, and less room for error, support and trust, thus perpetuating the cycle of oppression.

Unlike targets of oppression (Box 11.1), people in dominant groups are frequently unaware that they are members of the dominant group.

Box 11.1 **Oppression definitions.**

Oppression: The interaction of prejudice and institutional power results in a system that discriminates against groups known as 'non-dominant' groups, whilst benefiting others, referred to as 'dominant groups.'

Racism, sexism, ableism, classism and ageism are examples of oppressions which allow dominant groups to exert control over non-dominant groups by restricting their rights, freedoms and access to basic resources such as healthcare, education, employment and housing (the social determinants of healthcare) (see Chapter 4).

Internalised oppression: This is the process by which people in the non-dominant group internalise and personalise oppression

---

by believing that prejudices and stereotypes about them are true (see Chapter 2). Internalised oppression occurs when members of non-dominant groups change their attitudes, behaviours, speech and self-confidence to reflect the dominant group's stereotypes and norms. Internalised oppression can lead to low self-esteem, self-doubt and, in extreme cases, self-loathing. Fear, criticism and distrust of one's non-dominant group members can also be projected outward.

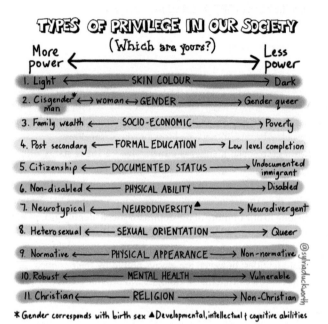

Figure 11.1 Types of privilege in our society. Depending on our social identity, certain privileges come with those identities. Depending on what value society places on that privilege comes more or less power. Source: © Sylvia Duckworth.

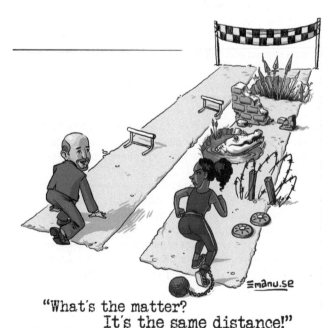

"What's the matter? It's the same distance!"

Figure 11.2 'Equality Race'. Source: © Emanu Garnheim.

Some privileges are visible, e.g. skin colour, body size and physical ability. Often, privilege operates in an unconscious way, invisible to those who have it (Figure 11.2). Peggy McIntosh described White privilege as an 'invisible weightless knapsack of special provisions, maps, passports, codebooks, visa, clothes, tools and blank checks' [2].

In healthcare settings, the constellation of personal and institutional privilege provides opportunities to either sustain racial healthcare privilege gaps or transform organisations and those who work within them to reduce healthcare inequalities effectively [3,4]. Put simply, privilege lets you live longer and healthier lives. Part of the process of becoming an ally (see Chapter 12) involves exploring and understanding how privilege operates in our own lives.

Power

'Power in defence of freedom is greater than power on behalf of tyranny and oppression, because power, real power, comes from our conviction which produces action, uncompromising action.'

(Malcolm X)

Power is a health and social justice (i.e. ensuring that there is fair and equitable division of resources, opportunities and privileges in society) issue. Although power has long been accepted as shaping people's lives, it is difficult to describe what it is and how it affects us. Yet increasingly, evidence tells us that power has a real effect on our health and wellbeing [5,6]. But what is our privilege and power (Box 11.2)?

Box 11.2 **Reflective exercises about privilege and power.**

Privilege
1. Review Figure 11.1; what privileges do you have?
2. Are these privileges visible or hidden?
3. Were you aware of these privileges?
4. Imagine yourself outside the group (or groups) where you currently belong:
   • What would you lose if you no longer belonged to that group (those groups)?
   • What would you gain?

Power
You have more influence over decisions that affect your life if you have power. When you can do this, it appears normal, and you are probably unaware of your own power. On the other hand, those with limited power may feel their voice goes unheard, and they have little control over important things.

If someone asked you to describe what it is to have power, what would you say? Having influence? Money? Knowledge?

If you think about the inequalities in power between people, what comes to mind? Oppression? Privilege? Disadvantage? What do these concepts mean in the context of health?

Power is 'the ability to decide who will access resources; the capacity to direct or influence the behaviour of others, oneself, and/or the course of events'. Power doesn't belong to one person but exists in the relationships between individuals and groups of people. Like privilege, power is also context specific: people can have a lot of power in some situations but can be powerless in others.

The power that we hold is intricately linked to the privileges that we have (Figure 11.3).

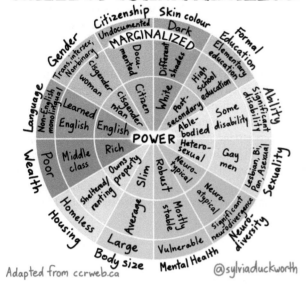

Figure 11.3 Wheel of power and privilege. This illustration shows how powerful personal and social identities are. Those people with minimal power are often marginalised members of our society.
Source: © Sylvia Duckworth.

Alongside income and wealth, unequal distribution of power across the population is one of the fundamental causes of health inequalities (see Chapter 4). In a classic study, Steven Lukes [7] demonstrated that coercive power can take covert forms. Power manifests itself, for example, in the ability of advantaged groups to shape the agenda of public debate and decision making in such a way that disadvantaged members of society are denied a voice. At a deeper societal level, dominant groups can shape people's perceptions and preferences; for example, by controlling the mass media, they can gaslight the oppressed to believe they have no serious grievances.

The World Health Organization describes four different types of power [8].

1 'Power *over*' is when someone or some people are able to influence or coerce others. This can be the most negative form of power.
2 'Power *to*' is where individuals are able to organise or change existing hierarchies or structures.
3 'Power *with*' is the collective power of communities or organisations.
4 'Power *within*' is each individual's capacity to exercise control or act on their own will.

The impact of power on health inequalities

Power, or lack thereof, can significantly impact people's circumstances and control over things that affect them, such as their health. Individuals may have fewer options, are unable to make informed decisions and as a result, may not receive the healthcare services they require (Box 11.3). It is widely accepted that power must be distributed more evenly for

everyone's health and wellbeing. This entails empowering disadvantaged communities and groups to have greater control over the factors influencing their health [6].

> **Box 11.3 No privilege and no power.**
>
> Imani Alexander, 38 years old, is Black and suffers from bipolar disorder. She was hospitalised due to severe abdominal pain. She struggled to walk due to the pain she was in and arrived at the Accident and Emergency department in a wheelchair with her husband. On arrival, the receptionist rolled her eyes when Imani explained that she was in severe pain and 'needed something' to ease her pain. The receptionist asked that she get out of the wheelchair so that 'someone who actually needs it can use it'. Imani tried to explain that she was struggling to walk due to the pain but acceded to the request. After a several-hour wait, she was assessed by a Dr Armitage who stated that as her observations were normal, she 'can't be in that much pain' and that he would prescribe some paracetamol and ibuprofen for her pending her blood test results being reviewed. Whilst waiting, Imani's pain increased, and she became very distressed, asking for stronger pain relief. Dr Armitage returned and dismissed her pain by saying, 'you need to calm down!'. Imani clinically deteriorated and was subsequently diagnosed with a ruptured appendix.
>
> In addition to her race and gender, Imani also had the added marginalised identity of having a diagnosed psychiatric condition. Racism in patient care is well documented and there is a plethora of data which demonstrates the discriminatory experiences of Black patients. Black women are often caught between being considered impervious to pain because of their race but overly hysterical because of their gender. Black patients are 22% less likely than White patients to receive appropriate pain relief (see Chapter 3). In this situation, there are multiple marginalised identities that mean that Imani is dismissed by healthcare team members and also lacks the privileges and power that she needs in order to advocate for herself to optimise her outcome.

Intersectionality

'Intersectionality is a lens through which you can see where power comes and collides, where it locks and intersects. It is the acknowledgement that everyone has their own unique experiences of discrimination and privilege'

(Kimberlé Crenshaw)

Intersectionality is a theory of social relations (Box 11.4) that examines intersecting forms of identities. It entails acknowledging that social systems are complicated and that multiple forms of oppression and prejudice, such as racism, sexism and ageism, may be present and active in a person's life simultaneously.

> **Box 11.4 History of intersectionality.**
>
> Intersectionality originates in the Black feminist movement, with legal scholar Kimberlé Crenshaw coining the term. Crenshaw

believed that both the anti-racist and feminist movements ignored the unique challenges that Black women face. She stated that legislation concerning race is intended to protect Black men, whereas legislation concerning sexism protects White women. As a result, simply combining racism and sexism does not protect Black women.

Intersectional theory is now being applied to a variety of social and healthcare issues, as well as contributing to an increased understanding of dominant identities such as those associated with Whiteness, masculinity and heterosexuality. Intersectionality encompasses more than having multiple identities; it is not a simple solution to equality and diversity issues. It is, however, a necessary framework as we truly engage with work to bring issues of privilege and power into the open to gain health and social equity.

Source: Crenshaw, K. (1989) *Demarginalizing the Intersection of Race and Sex: A Black Feminist Critique of Antidiscrimination Doctrine, Feminist Theory and Antiracist Politics*. Chicago: University of Chicago Legal Forum.

Intersectionality promotes an understanding of humans as being shaped by the interaction of different social identities, e.g. race, ethnicity, gender, class, sexuality, geography, age, disability/ability, migration status and religion (Figure 11.4). These interactions occur within a context of connected systems and structures of power, e.g. law, policies, state governments, religious institutions and media. Through such processes, interdependent forms of privilege and oppression shaped by colonialism, imperialism, racism, homophobia, ableism and patriarchy are created [9]. Intersectionality is concerned with the ways in which multiple social identities intersect with one another at the macro- (national and international), meso- (regional institutions and policies) and micro- (community, grassroots and individual) levels.

At its core, intersectionality is about understanding and addressing *all* potential roadblocks to an individual or group's wellbeing. However, it is critical to understand that it is not as simple as adding up the oppressions and addressing each one separately. 'Isms' such as racism, sexism, xenophobia, classism and ableism exist on their own. However, those 'isms' *compound*, *transform* and *amplify* the experience of oppression for underprivileged and powerless members of society (Figure 11.5).

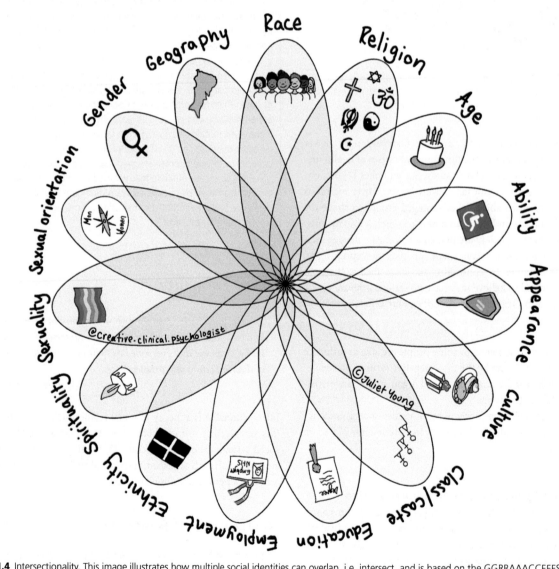

Figure 11.4 Intersectionality. This image illustrates how multiple social identities can overlap, i.e. intersect, and is based on the GGRRAAACCEEESSS model by Burnham [10].
Source: © Dr Juliet Young, clinical psychologist. Permission granted for use within this book.

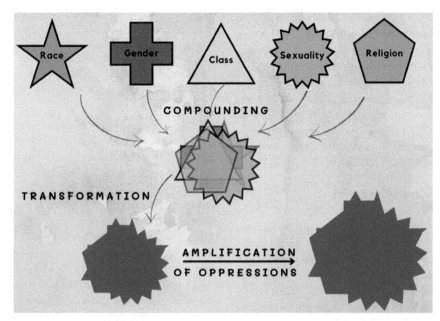

Figure 11.5 Compounding, transformation and amplification of intersectional identities. Intersectionality refers to the inseparable ways in which each non-dominant component of our identity intersects and transforms to amplify discriminatory practices or power imbalances and oppression towards an individual. The oppression that an individual experiences often reflects a lack of privileges and power. When considering intersectionality, it is key to understand that it is not simply a layering effect of multiple identities. Every visible and invisible, non-dominant social identity *compounds* those marginalised identities and *transforms* them to make a whole new identity. This intersectional identity can cause an *amplification* of the oppression that people with intersectionality can experience. (The shape chosen for each identity is arbitrary and not a reflection of the subcategories of that specific social identity.) Source: © Dr Shehla Imtiaz-Umer.

Going beyond the definition of intersectionality to unpack its fundamental tenets is critical (Table 11.1). It considers that while a young, White, able-bodied, heterosexual woman's career may improve with gender equality initiatives, it may not be of any significant benefit to an older, Black, disabled lesbian – she will continue to have her progress in the workplace and wider society hampered by racism, ableism and homophobia. Intersectionality allows us to understand how nuances in social positioning affect individuals' healthcare access and outcomes.

By understanding intersectionality, we can shift our thinking from frameworks that benefit dominant identities to frameworks that are mindful of the prejudices faced by our colleagues and patients and how their social identities contribute to their experience of the world. We can listen to others, examine our own privileges and ask questions about who may be excluded from the space we are in or adversely affected by the work we are doing. More importantly, it means taking measurable action to invite, include and centre the voices and work of marginalised individuals (see Chapters 12 and 13).

Intersectionality and health

To understand why discrimination is important for health, consider the role of social institutions such as schools, hospitals and the legal system in controlling populations. They have control over who enters and what experiences they have there. Children from lower-income families are underrepresented among university students, while Black men are overrepresented in prisons. Discrimination in the criminal justice system, education system, healthcare system and society at large is a significant reason for such disparities.

Table 11.1 Tenets of intersectionality.

Intersectionality tenet	
Human lives and not single categories	Be aware that humans cannot be distilled into single categories based on the identities they have
No predetermination	The importance of any category or social category cannot be predetermined. It is context specific
Multi-level analysis	This links individual experiences to broader structures and systems of power across time and space
Simultaneous privilege and oppression	Traditionally, marginalised groups are not homogeneous and as such, people can experience concurrent privilege and oppression. For example, a White man who is a wheelchair user will have the privilege of his White male identity but will be oppressed due to his physical disability
Self-reflexivity	It is necessary to understand how one's own privilege and/or oppression positions operate within an intra- and interpersonal context
Social justice	Any work done in or on intersectionality from a research policy or practice must be oriented towards social justice

Source: Based on Lancet Commission on Gender and Global Health. Intersectionality & Reflections on Gender and Global Health. www.youtube.com/watch?v=cxMlzIabLac 2021

When considering health inequalities, the historical approach has been to address a single issue at a time, e.g. gender inequality or race inequality. However, adopting this single-axis analysis of inequalities experienced by patients results in a limited, one-dimensional and incomplete understanding of health inequality. Intersectionality has received little attention from researchers and public health professionals thus far but we are now seeing signs that it is being taken seriously [9,11,12]. The COVID-19 pandemic accelerated the focus on and understanding of the role of intersectionality in analysing who lives, who works, who dies and who thrives [13].

Intersectionality in clinical practice

Consideration of the application of intersectionality specifically to the clinical medicine setting has primarily focused on specific groups of individuals rather than its broad applicability. While the impact of health inequalities is being extensively researched, there appears to be a lack of the same dynamism to understand the impact of intersectionality on health inequalities. Despite advancements in diagnostic technology, diagnostic errors and delays continue to cause significant physical and psychological harm to patients and financial harm to the healthcare system [14]. Some of these misdiagnoses are caused by systemic biases that disproportionately affect historically marginalised groups because of their intersectional identities.

The use of intersectionality in clinical practice enables clinicians to be as knowledgeable about their patients' sociodemographic characteristics as they are about the pathobiology of their symptoms and illness (Box 11.5).

Individual differences in social class and education highlight structural issues that cannot be directly changed in the clinical encounter, but clinicians can assist patients in receiving resources that can improve health outcomes by paying attention to the social determinants of health that intersectionality highlights.

Using intersectionality in clinical encounters allows us to gain insight into how thinking from an intersectional framework can enrich patient–clinician encounters, increase patient-centredness and aid in navigating better clinical experiences.

Intersectionality in research and policy development

While the clinician–patient interaction is a micro-level interaction, the interaction does not occur in a vacuum. Instead, social categories interact with and reinforce one another. With this in mind, it is essential to consider how broader institutions and policies influence and are influenced by our social identities, shaping those clinician–patient interactions.

When considering how to address health inequities, the goal of any intersectionality-focused intervention should be based on precise informed analysis that would allow targeted and more effective policy and programme development. Currently, there is no single way to approach intersectionality analyses in health research and policy. However, there are fundamental principles which researchers could apply to ensure that the needs of as many people as possible are being met on a meso- and macro-level (Box 11.6) [15].

Box 11.5 **Intersectionality in chronic pain.**

Aminul Miah is a 42-year-old factory worker. English is his second language. He has had several phone consultations regarding his back pain. He has been given paracetamol, ibuprofen and naproxen, and has been referred to the physiotherapist but the pain has not settled. He has been booked in with Dr Holliday.

Aminul is calling today to ask for stronger analgesia to manage his pain. During the appointment, he explains that the physiotherapist sent him 'a link or something' on his phone to do some exercises, but he struggled to follow the instructions. His manager at the factory has said that if he goes off work 'sick' then his pay will be deducted. Aminul is unsure what to do as he can't work but also can't afford to be off work. Dr Holliday asks why he didn't do the exercises and rebukes him for not just 'following the videos'. He also tells him that he 'can't have anything stronger' because he 'didn't even bother doing the exercises' that the physiotherapist sent him, before ending the consultation.

Ethnic minority people are overrepresented in physically demanding jobs such as factory workers, cleaners and construction workers, making their jobs a common source of injury and chronic pain. Intersectionality demonstrates that one's class status may be more pertinent in some contexts than others.

The patient's social identity is clearly not the issue. Rather, the issue is how patients are marginalised as a result of discriminatory social and structural practices because of their intersectional identity. Inattention to the patient's intersecting social identities and how social structures reinforce disadvantage leads to further marginalisation.

Box 11.6 **How to incorporate intersectionality analyses into health research.**

Conceptualising the research
- What and who is being studied?
- Who is being compared and why? What assumptions underlie these choices?
- What new issues of disadvantage, privilege and resistance or agency are addressed by the research?

Designing the study
- Is there adequate information on the aspects of the social location of the study population?
  - Is there disaggregated data by sex, ethnicity, class and other categories?
  - What processes may determine their health?
- Do these considerations inform the selection of a population to capture diverse experiences?
- Who is excluded?
- How will the research capture dynamic interactions between multiple health-influencing factors rather than simple additions?

Interpretation and impact
- How will commonalities and differences within and across population groups be recognised without being reductionistic or universalising categories and cultures?
- Does the analysis link interactions at individual levels of experience to social institutions and processes, broader structures of power and historical or contemporary patterns of inequality? What are the implications of the research for reducing inequities and advancing global health goals?

Source: Kapilashrami and Hankivsky [15].

Evidence for the positive outcomes of applying an intersectionality framework exists. Conducting such research is difficult and time-consuming at each stage of the research process [16] but the knowledge gained justifies this new approach to health inequalities work. Unequivocally incorporating intersectionality into health research is not only possible but can also make significant contributions to reducing health and social inequity [17].

Impact of intersectionality on medical education

Western medicine and medical institutions are embedded within power structures that favour White, cisgender and heterosexual men (see Chapter 7). Dismantling power structures in medicine requires the same complex thinking as considering intersectionality in our patient populations. For example, medical textbooks reinforce Whiteness norms by underrepresenting racial and ethnic minorities. Examining exclusion and discrimination in medical education, training and workplace experiences is the first step toward recognising systemic, intersecting inequities in professional medical culture (see Chapter 5). For example, a White woman may experience a relative advantage over a Black man during medical selection and training. But it is also true that neither White women nor Black men are homogeneous in their experiences of advantage or disadvantage (see Chapter 6). There is, however, increased recognition of the importance of diversifying the curricula to reflect the communities we serve to ensure health equity *and* social equity (see Chapter 13).

Intersectionality in the healthcare workforce

Abundant data illustrate the disparity in healthcare workforce experiences – affecting nurses, doctors, medical students, management and other non-clinical staff (see Chapter 3). Traditionally, this has been disproportionately attributed to race or gender. The 2022 BMA report had a section specifically outlining the prejudices faced by staff due to their intersectional identities (Box 11.7). These experiences highlight the importance of using an intersectionality lens to understand and address how discrimination within the workforce manifests.

Box 11.7 **Intersectionality in the BMA Racism in Medicine report.**

Thirty percent of respondents thought that the racism they experienced was linked to religion and belief, with many respondents mentioning Islamophobic, Antisemitic or other faith-based slurs and discrimination.
- 'Not allowing Muslims a prayer space – it literally takes 5–10 minutes to pray, this does not affect my job as a doctor … is a key factor putting me off certain careers in medicine.' (Medical student, Bangladeshi, England)
- 'People seem to exhibit cognitive dissonance … they accept overt racism towards people of colour is wrong, but somehow do not apply the same standard to anti-Jewish racism.' (Consultant, White British, England)

Over a quarter of respondents (28%) reported that experiences of racism were exacerbated by sex, with many women describing instances in which they had been degraded and belittled.
- 'Racist remarks from delirious elderly patients. Racism associated with sexism – the assumption of not being a real doctor due to being an Asian female.' (Junior doctor, Asian British, England)

The intersection of ethnicity, religion and gender was evident in comments from respondents who wore headscarves. They described discriminatory policies and behaviours that made it more difficult for them to practise medicine while wearing a headscarf.
- 'Being removed from emergency operating theatre by a senior ODP/ theatre manager who took offence to my headscarf, could not provide a head covering that would fit over it.' (Locally employed doctor, Asian, England)
- 'Not being able to wear a theatre hijab in theatre without a disposable cap on top which truly makes no sense.' (Medical student, Pakistani, England)

Source: BMA (2022) Racism in Medicine. www.bma.org.uk/media/5746/bma-racism-in-medicine-survey-report-15-june-2022.pdf

---

There have been highly publicised and prominent regulatory cases within the medical workforce that can be attributed to intersectionality (Box 11.8) and see Further resources.

Box 11.8 **Dr Hadiza Bawa-Garba – power, privilege and intersectionality in the NHS.**

An ST6* with an 'impeccable record', Dr Bawa-Garba had returned from maternity leave and was on her first acute medical shift on that fateful day of 18th February 2011. The case of the tragic death of Jack Adcock and subsequent criminal and regulatory charges against Dr Bawa-Garba garnered international attention and is well documented through various legal, regulatory, procedural and media reports which are widely available.

After the criminal trial resulted in a two-year suspended sentence (appeal quashed), the Medical Practitioners Tribunal Service (MPTS) decided to suspend the paediatric trainee for 12 months for her indirect role in Jack's death. However, the General Medical Council (GMC) – the public body that regulates doctors in the UK – fought to appeal the initial tribunal decision, which led to Dr Bawa-Garba being erased from the medical register for UK doctors. The subsequent outcry by medical professionals for the unfair treatment and scapegoating of Dr Bawa-Garba, in the context of multiple systemic issues, resulted in grassroots support which crowdfunded her subsequent legal appeals. She won those appeals and was added back to the GMC register in order to complete her paediatric training. In 2022 she was appointed as a consultant.

Of particular note is that Dr Bawa-Garba is a female Nigerian who wears the hijab. This intersectional identity was heavily politicised in media articles – subjecting her to racist, Islamophobic and misogynistic contempt. There were ongoing concerns that had her race, gender and faith been different, she would not have been scapegoated in this case as she was.

Additionally, her consultant, Dr Stephen O'Riordan, a White, male senior clinician, had been advised of the same blood results and did not review Jack. Dr O'Riordan subsequently relocated to Ireland where he continues to practise and having been deregistered by the GMC at his own request, did not have his involvement scrutinised.

Reviewing this case through the lens of privilege, power, and intersectionality, it can be seen as an example of White, male privilege.

Dr O'Riordan had power through his seniority and social identities, thus granting him privileges which contrast with Dr Bawa-Garba's marginalised identities and the prejudiced experiences that she faced.
(*ST6 denotes 6th year of specialist training)

Sources: BBC News. The struck off doctor. www.bbc.co.uk/news/resources/idt-sh/the_struck_off_doctor (Accessed 15 October 2022)
Pulse Today. Bawa-Garba – timeline of a case that has rocked medicine. www.pulsetoday.co.uk/analysis/regulation/bawa-garba-timeline-of-a-case-that-has-rocked-medicine (accessed 15 October 2022)

Intersectionality and allyship

Allyship is as multifaceted as intersectionality and becomes even more important when considering that an individual can have both privileged and marginalised identities. In any situation of oppression which requires allyship, regardless of an individual's concurrent marginalised identity, their privileged identity will also be present (see Chapter 12). Self-reflexivity is needed to understand the impact of those privileged identities in a context where oppression or prejudice is occurring [18].

Redistributing power

Patients

Those who work for public bodies have a vital role in ensuring that their operations are equitable. The available resources and opportunities, particularly for disadvantaged groups, should enable communities to have greater control. In the UK, legislated changes to delivering healthcare have resulted in the formation of statutory organisations called integrated care boards (ICB) and integrated care systems (ICS). By bringing the NHS together locally to improve population health and establish shared strategic priorities within the NHS, this new structure aims to facilitate proactive and positive engagement with communities to place their views at the heart of policy and healthcare delivery decision making.

These new structures need to be utilised to ensure that rather than being directed by those already holding positions of power, policy makers and service providers should actively and respectfully engage, involve and empower disadvantaged communities [5].

Workforce

Report after report has highlighted the differential experiences of healthcare workers. There is recognition that cultural transformation is needed across all aspects of the NHS (see Further resources) and the healthcare systems including selection, attainment, individual experiences and staff diversity. A whole-systems approach is necessary to address the systemic, pervasive nature of oppression and prejudice due to intersectionality that causes a toxic environment for too many colleagues. What can we do to shift the power?

- Move from data gathering/reporting to affirmative action.
- Ensure senior visible, diverse leadership and role models.
- Provide a robust, anonymous reporting mechanism to avoid fears of retribution and overcome barriers to reporting.
- Support those who experience discriminatory behaviours from colleagues/patients.

- Have accountability from leaders who fail act on the data within their workplace showing persistent discriminatory experiences.

Conclusion

Although tasked with serving all people, healthcare systems tend to project values and provide services that meet the needs of the majority while not fully recognising the needs of the minority. Leadership positions in the healthcare system are occupied mainly by individuals of privilege and enabled by their social identities, including race. This same system then tends to provide services that meet the needs of the dominant group while not fully recognising the needs of the non-dominant groups who continue to face prejudice and oppression. Traditionally, there have been single-axis interventions to overcome barriers to healthcare. Although there appears to be an increased focus on the role of intersectionality in ensuring social and health equity, much more needs to be done in the face of innumerable challenges.

Further reading/resources

BBC News. The struck off doctor. www.bbc.co.uk/news/resources/idt-sh/the_struck_off_doctor (accessed 15 October 2022)

BMA (2022) Delivering racial equality in medicine. www.bma.org.uk/media/5745/bma-delivering-racial-equality-in-medicine-report-15-june-2022.pdf (accessed 15 October 2022)

BMA. A fight for fairness beating discrimination. www.bma.org.uk/news-and-opinion/a-fight-for-fairness-beating-racial-discrimination#:~:text=The%20GMC%20is%20appealing%20the,compared%20differed%20in%20key%20respects (accessed 15 October 2022)

BMA (2022) Racism in medicine. www.bma.org.uk/media/5746/bma-racism-in-medicine-survey-report-15-june-2022.pdf (Accessed 15 October 2022)

Crenshaw, K. (1989) *Demarginalizing the Intersection of Race and Sex: A Black Feminist Critique of Antidiscrimination Doctrine, Feminist Theory and Antiracist Politics*. Chicago: University of Chicago Legal Forum.

Kar, P. (2022) Manjula Arora case: the GMC stumbles again? *BMJ*, **377**, o1327.

Liu, E. (2014) How to understand power. TED-Ed Talks. www.youtube.com/watch?v=c_Eutci7ack (accessed 5 October 2022)

McDonald, P. and Vaughan, J. (2018) The aftermath of the Sellu case for law and the medical profession. *RCS Bulletin*. https://publishing.rcseng.ac.uk/doi/pdf/10.1308/rcsbull.2018.207 (accessed 25 October 2022)

Medical Practitioners Tribunal Service. Dr. Manjula Arora. www.mpts-uk.org/hearings-and-decisions/medical-practitioners-tribunals/mrs-manjula-arora-may-22 (accessed 21 October 2022)

NHS England. We are the NHS: People Plan 2020/21 – Action for Us All, 2021. www.england.nhs.uk/wp-content/uploads/2020/07/We-Are-The-NHS-Action-For-All-Of-Us-FINAL-March-21.pdf (Accessed 30 September 2022)

Pulse Today. Bawa-Garba – timeline of a case that has rocked medicine. www.pulsetoday.co.uk/analysis/regulation/bawa-garba-timeline-of-a-case-that-has-rocked-medicine (accessed 15 October 2022)

References

1 Tajfel, H. and Turner, J.C. (2004) *The Social Identity Theory of Intergroup Behavior*. New York: Psychology Press

2 McIntosh, P. (2019) White privilege: unpacking the invisible knapsack (1989). In: *On Privilege, Fraudulence, and Teaching as Learning*. New York: Routledge.

3 Hobbs, J. (2018) White privilege in health care: following recognition with action. *Annals of Family Medicine*, **16** (3), 197–198.

4 Romano, M.J. (2018) White privilege in a white coat: how racism shaped my medical education. *Annals of Family Medicine*, **16** (3), 261–263.

5 Dickie, E., Hearty, W., Fraser, A. et al. (2015) Power – a health and social justice issue. www.healthscotland.scot/media/2205/power-a-health-and-social-justice-issue.pdf

6 NHS Scotland. (2015) Health inequalities: what are they? How do we reduce them? www.healthscotland.scot/media/1086/health-inequalities-what-are-they-how-do-we-reduce-them-mar16.pdf

7 Lukes, S. (2004) *Power: A Radical View*, 2e. Basingstoke: Palgrave Macmillan.

8 World Health Organization (2010) A conceptual framework for action on the social determinants of health. https://apps.who.int/iris/handle/10665/44489

9 Hankivsky, O., Grace, D., Hunting, G. et al. (2014) An intersectionality-based policy analysis framework: critical reflections on a methodology for advancing equity. *International Journal of Equity in Health*, **13** (1), 119.

10 Burnham, J. (2012) Developments in Social GRRRAAACCEEESSS: visible–invisible and voiced–unvoiced 1. In: Krause, I.B. *Culture and Reflexivity in Systemic Psychotherapy*. Oxford: Routledge.

11 Samra, R. and Hankivsky, O. (2021) Adopting an intersectionality framework to address power and equity in medicine. *Lancet*, **397** (10277), 857–859.

12 Holman, D., Salway, S., Bell, A. et al. (2021) Can intersectionality help with understanding and tackling health inequalities? Perspectives of professional stakeholders. *Health Research Policy and Systems*, **19** (1), 97.

13 Bowleg, L. (2020) We're not all in this together: on COVID-19, intersectionality, and structural inequality. *American Journal of Public Health*, **110** (7), 917.

14 Khullar, D., Jha, A.K. and Jena, A.B. (2015) Reducing diagnostic errors – why now? *New England Journal of Medicine*, **373** (26), 2491–2493.

15 Kapilashrami, A. and Hankivsky, O. (2018) Intersectionality and why it matters to global health. *Lancet*, **391** (10140), 2589–2591.

16 Yam, E.A., Silva, M., Ranganathan, M. et al. (2021) Time to take critical race theory seriously: moving beyond a colour-blind gender lens in global health. *Lancet Global Health*, **9** (4), e389–390.

17 Hankivsky, O., Doyal, L., Einstein, G. et al. (2017) The odd couple: using biomedical and intersectional approaches to address health inequities. *Global Health Action*, **10** (sup2), 1326686.

18 Understanding intersectionality and engaging with diverse staff and communities. NHS Employers. www.nhsemployers.org/articles/understanding-intersectionality-and-engaging-diverse-staff-and-communities.

CHAPTER 12

Allyship and Being an 'Active Bystander'

Diana Lautenberger

Director, Gender Equity Initiatives, Academic Affairs, Association of American Medical Colleges, Washington, DC, USA

OVERVIEW

- Allyship is a life-long relationship built on trust and solidarity where the ally actively uses their privilege to change harmful patterns of injustices.
- Individuals must explore and acknowledge their privilege(s), background and positionality in developing their allyship skills.
- Those working in solidarity as allies should be conscious of avoiding performative allyship.
- Intervention during harmful situations, or being an active bystander, is one action of allyship.
- Bystander intervention or 'active bystanders' recognise potentially harmful situations and choose to act and intervene in a way that can positively impact the outcome.
- Organisations should embed allyship and active bystander intervention strategies by creating community agreements that establish an accountability culture rewarded by leadership.

Allyship

Wherever you are in your allyship journey – either your first day or already an experienced ally – starting the journey is the most crucial step. Becoming an ally means honestly facing your privileges and identities (Chapter 11), which can be challenging. Allyship is important for many reasons, particularly given the positive impact on individuals [1]. However, organisations also benefit from allyship. Culture change occurs little by little when people choose to step up and challenge oppressive norms and culture. Many think that general well-intentioned attitudes will eventually change things over time. This passive approach to justice and equity is why we have not yet made enough progress. Systems of inequality are so ingrained and strong that they won't change unless individuals intentionally and actively start resetting cultural norms.

Allyship is one way to do this. The act of challenging these norms won't be so uncomfortable if more people step up. Audre Lorde eloquently noted, 'The master's tools won't dismantle the master's house'.

These concepts and topics are complex. There isn't always one straightforward correct answer. Readers may be inclined to dissect these concepts and find contradictions. Sometimes there are contradictions. It is essential to resist the urge to put things neatly in boxes because this work requires complex relational exploration, emotions and action. Most of all, allyship restores us to our humanity – when we fight for justice and equity in our communities, we restore our whole selves with love, respect and wellbeing.

What is allyship?

The terms 'ally' and 'allyship' have existed for some time and have been integral to the fight for equity and justice. There isn't a single definition, but many. Helpful definitions describe the foundational elements and behaviours of allies (Box 12.1).

> Box 12.1 **Foundational elements and behaviours of allies.**
>
> Allies are people who recognize the unearned privilege they receive from society's patterns of injustice and take responsibility for changing these patterns [1].
>
> A lifelong process of building relationships based on trust, consistency, and accountability with marginalised individuals and/or groups of people [2].
>
> Allyship is a strategic mechanism used by individuals to become collaborators, accomplices, and co-conspirators who fight injustice and promote equity in the workplace through supportive personal relationships and public acts of sponsorship and advocacy [3].

What these definitions uncover are three foundational elements of allyship.

1 Allyship is inherently active; it cannot be passive.
2 An ally is continually working on themselves, starting by recognising their privilege(s).
3 Allyship is inherently uncomfortable.

Allyship can be uncomfortable because you are actively confronting and interrogating systems of oppression and dominant cultures. Therefore, if you aren't uncomfortable, at least sometimes, you may not be practising allyship authentically (Box 12.2).

ABC of Equality, Diversity and Inclusion in Healthcare, First Edition. Edited by Shehla Imtiaz-Umer and John Frain.
© 2023 John Wiley & Sons Ltd. Published 2023 by John Wiley & Sons Ltd.

> **Box 12.2 'Visible but comfortable' isn't allyship.**
>
> Jane is a colleague who actively refers to herself as an ally when conversations around diversity, equity and inclusion or social justice conversations come up. Her department has had a few town halls (meetings) to discuss racial justice issues. She is always a vocal proponent of supporting Black, Indigenous and People of Colour (BIPOC) communities. During the racial justice uprisings of 2020, she put a "Black Lives Matter" sign on her office door and encouraged conversation with other White and dominant-identity colleagues. Jane is attending a research committee meeting for a new faculty member. The research committee chair, with whom Jane is friends, opens up the discussion by saying, 'Okay, we do need to recruit more diverse faculty, but I don't want to lower our standards so if the person ends up being a woman or a person of colour, great, but let's keep our options open'. Jane says nothing.

Another way to reflect on allyship is if the marginalised group you're trying to align yourself with wouldn't call you an ally, you probably aren't practising allyship. Only those we are trying to align ourselves with in solidarity and support can truly say whether we are allies – it's not something we can necessarily self-define, and it is not an identity.

Allyship is a process (Figure 12.1) and begins with understanding our own identities and which of these identities may have more or less privilege. It is then up to the ally that they actively stand up for others to interrupt harmful behaviours. Finally, the individual should receive feedback from others if their allyship is effective and supportive or furthering harm.

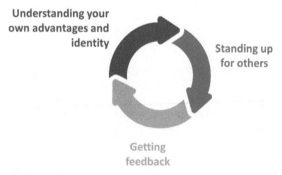

Understanding your own advantages and identity

Standing up for others

Getting feedback

Figure 12.1 The process of allyship. This continuous feedback cycle allows allies to reflect further and start the process again. It is important to recognise that allyship is a life-long continuous relationship-building exercise in collaboration with others we want to support. Ultimately, the aim is to redefine the cultural norms in our organisations so that they are equitable and inclusive.

Intersectionality and allyship

Allyship can be considered through the lens of intersectionality. Intersectionality becomes critical in allyship practice because many of us have privileged *and* marginalised identities (see Chapter 11). Those with both privileged and marginalised identities must be actively aware of these identities in each situation and opportunity for allyship [2]. This may be referred to as one's positionality in allyship.

For example, a gay, White woman may experience sexism and homophobia oppression (Box 12.3). Still, in a situation that requires their allyship as a White person, they must be hyperaware that they are bringing this identity into every situation – regardless of their marginalised ones.

> **Box 12.3 Not equating experiences.**
>
> Alice is an openly gay, White, cis-gendered woman who has been at the hospital for 15 years. In a departmental meeting, a male senior clinician continually interrupts the only Black woman clinician in the department, Renee. He talks over her, and everyone can see she is becoming visibly upset but no one intervenes. After the meeting, a group of colleagues stay behind to chat and console Renee. Alice walks over and expresses her frustration, 'I can't believe that guy; it's so frustrating for us to go through this every day. I completely understand what you're going through; he says anti-queer stuff to me all the time. I'm going to write a letter to the head of the department!' In this situation, Alice is trying to equate her experience of oppression as a gay woman to that of a Black woman, which is a different experience since she is also White. She is centring herself at this moment and not staying aware of her White identity, taking up space in the room when harm has just happened to Renee. She also centres herself by recommending she write a letter after the fact instead of intervening in the moment to support Renee.

For those allies with an intersectional identity, being an ally to some groups can inevitably be more comfortable due to shared lived experiences in comparison to other groups of people, where the allyship journey must start from the beginning.

While these are some standard definitions of allyship, it's important when developing allyship education and programmes that institutions actively involve marginalised individuals in developing and expressing their allyship frameworks.

Those with dominant identities must listen to experts and experiences of marginalisation and support, and not dominate allyship work as part of an overall diversity, equity and inclusion strategy.

How can we be allies?

Allyship is as much about an in-the-moment intervention as it is about continual reflection and unlearning. There are several ways in which allies can engage meaningfully in their commitment to support others and radically challenge systems of oppression and inequity [3].

- *Accept that you will make mistakes.* We are bound to not get it right along the way in any life-long process. Most importantly, we do not pull back after these mistakes but always choose to re-engage. We have a cultural tendency to avoid situations where we may fail, so actively fighting against these dominant cultural traits is critical.
- *Embrace discomfort and have uncomfortable conversations.* These are inherently uncomfortable conversations and situations, so we must lean into them. Our culture, especially in healthcare, does not often make space for complex emotions or emotions at all.
- *Acknowledging and openly discussing your privileges/advantages.* The first step allies can take on their solidarity journey is to discuss

their privileges (or social advantages) openly. Hence, they understand their positionality in every potential situation where they can be an ally.

- *Listening more and speaking less.* Those of us with dominant identities are used to having the social advantage to take up space – physically, verbally and emotionally. Being an ally means stepping back and allowing others airtime, listening to what marginalised groups and individuals are asking from you – if they're asking for anything at all.

- *Not expecting to be educated by marginalised group members.* Oppression has existed for all human history, but many are realising the extent of these oppressions for the first time. While it is a positive sign that many are curious to learn more, allies mustn't be looking to marginalised peers and friends to help with this education. There are many resources, books, articles, podcasts, etc. to do some initial learning and processing on our own.

- *Welcoming and accepting feedback as radical care.* When others are giving us feedback, especially challenging feedback, an initial response is to become defensive. Being an ally means suspending your automatic defensive responses to hear the perspectives of others. If someone is taking the time to give feedback, it's essential to listen and be open-minded, as it is crucial to recognise it as an act of love and care for the ally to do better.

- *Recognising our needs comes secondary to those we are working with as allies.* Many who are early in allyship journeys can be very excited to get to work and show that we are supportive of change. Sometimes that means we need to show others how much we know, that we're progressive or 'woke'. To be an authentic ally, our need to show our allyship or knowledge in this area is not prioritised over what the targeted person in that situation wants.

- *Not expecting awards or special recognition.* Motivations to act as an ally shouldn't come with the expectation of being recognised, getting a pat on the back or extra social credit.

Reflection question

Take a moment and think about the last section.

1 Which of these ways are you engaged in already?
2 Which of these ways are you still working on?
3 What is a barrier to engaging in any of these?

How can we do better at being allies?

Having explored some definitions of allyship, and described what it is and how it looks and feels, it's also important to talk about what it *isn't*. Allyship is not the same as being an active bystander, being a saviour, posting stickers or signs, only intervening when convenient for you, or because it will make you feel good. Most of all, allyship isn't – easy. Discussing how we might get allyship wrong is just as important. This raises the concept of performative allyship – which many well-meaning allies can fall into if they aren't staying vigilant in their solidarity against oppression.

Performative allyship is a term that describes individuals who want to be perceived as allies for social gain and so exhibit outwardly, or socially acceptable, activities related to allyship – but are not actively confronting their privilege or taking responsibility for

changing harmful patterns of oppression [4]. This type of allyship may look like putting up a Black Lives Matter sign on your window or reposting something on social media related to social justice movements. While these acts individually can be positive, if they are the *only* type of activity you are engaged in, this is a sign your allyship might be performative (Box 12.4).

Box 12.4 Is your allyship performative?

1 Are you actively speaking out against oppression continuously or only when it is a hot topic?
2 Are you actively calling people 'out/in' when they say harmful, biased or oppressive things?
3 Are you educating yourself by reading articles or books, or watching movies that educate you on privilege, oppression and equity movements – or did you stop after a few?
4 Have you done something in support of an equity movement that you didn't tell anyone about? Put another way: are you always publicly vocalising your allyship?

Developing allyship skills

From ally to accomplice and co-conspirator

Allyship concepts are changing all the time, and so are the terms to define it. Many are now using the terms 'accomplice' or 'co-conspirator' to better define allyship as active and inherently subversive since you are working to dismantle systemic oppression [5]. This evolution of terminology also recalls the idea that allyship is a journey with a continuum of experiences and motivations. Keith Edwards' model of allyship is beneficial for understanding the continuum of allyship and how our awareness, motivations and behaviours change as we learn and practise (Table 12.1) [6].

Allyship scholar and expert Dr Sunny Nakae offers a model to describe this individual paradigm shift in our allyship journey from the 'me' to 'we' (Table 12.2).

Finally, to push our thinking of what allyship is, we must confront how allyship has been positioned in our society and what more we can do to take on the struggle as dominant-identity individuals. Consider this quote from Sonya Renee Taylor:

'I don't want an ally. Because an ally means you came here to help me … How are *you* helping *me* solve the problem *you* caused? Why aren't *I* helping *you* solve the problem *you* caused? Why am I not the ally and you the actor? Why is Blackness the responsibility holder and Whiteness gets to be the helper?' [7]

Whiteness, patriarchy and other dominant cultures susceptible to saviourship

With performative allyship in mind, it's essential to address how those with dominant identities are susceptible to co-opting and negatively attempting to practise allyship. This is sometimes referred to as 'White or male saviours'. For example, many early-career women describe experiences with an older White man in their department or clinic who professes to be a supporter of women but is, in reality, patronising and career limiting in his actions to 'support' women (Box 12.5). These well-meaning but harm-doing actions must be discussed openly and honestly so those interested in being allies can do

Table 12.1 Aspiring ally identity development.

	Self-interest	Altruism	Social justice
Motivation (conscious)	I want to help this person I know and care about	How can I help them?	In the end, I'm helping myself as well
Motivation (unconscious)	Protect	Guilt/shame	Freedom for self and others from oppression
View	This poor person Outrage at a person	You poor people, I should help Guilt	We're all in this together Collective consciousness
Behaviour	Address direct harm, prevent this behaviour from occurring again Separate from marginalised group	Separate self from dominant group I want to be the good one helping Exception to the norm	Recognise losses for all groups Hold self accountable for education and change
Outlook	The immediate act, not systems Hero to the person I don't see colour Working over	Systems, not individuals 'Other' is victim of oppression Work to empower others with self at centre Rescuer of the 'other' Working for	See intersections of systems and people and aspire to change both Constantly revisiting privilege Decentring your privileged identities Working with
Action	Rescue Unsure exactly what to say or do I speak up when obvious or convenient	Orchestrate a complex, public fix or response to get recognition I have the answer I speak up because I don't want people to think I'm a bigot	Consistently work in partnership I'm listening I speak up because any form of oppression hurts me

The conceptual continuum model presented here uses motivation (both conscious and unconscious), views, behaviours and outlooks to frame the different approaches and challenges facing aspiring allies. This model can be used as a tool for critical self-reflection to identify where an individual may be in their allyship development journey and for guidance in developing other aspiring allies. The three levels of allyship, described as self-interest, altruism and social justice, can be viewed as incremental and developmental as a continuum as an individual starts and works to develop their ally skills, moving through the stages from "self-interest" to "social justice".

Source: Keith Edwards, Aspiring Social Justice Allyship Identity Development, 2022.

Table 12.2 Allyship perspective shift from 'me' to 'we'.

Me	We
I'm not responsible	I'm inherently responsible
If not directed at me, not my place	Every context I share is my place
Ignore	Understand
Blindness	Awareness
Telling	Asking
Hurrying through, ignoring	Pausing, paying attention
I don't care	I don't know
Talking after	Intervening during

This table describes the change from internally 'me' focused attitudes, perspectives and behaviours toward one's responsibility of intervening in situations of harm to one of 'we', where the collective community is inherently responsible for intervening in an open, aware and curious way. Internally 'me' focused approaches to potential intervention represent historical and current modes of being (e.g. being a bystander) versus taking responsibility for reducing harm (e.g. being an active bystander).

Source: Sunny Nakae, Sunshine Medical Education Consulting LLC©, 2019.

better. Just as allyship is seen as a continuum, so are our privileged identities and how far we have come in our self-reflection.

> **Box 12.5 Allyship is supporting, not saving.**
>
> John is the department chair and has an excellent reputation at the institution – always an innovative and supportive leader. He regularly attends the Women in Medicine events to make opening comments and provides ample funding to the department's Diversity, Equity and Inclusion (DEI) initiatives. He is most proud of his support of the new Centre for Women's Advancement within the institution and takes every opportunity to discuss it. At the Centre's first anniversary celebration, he was supposed to make five minutes of comments but instead talked for 20 minutes about how important women's leadership is when the president of the Centre, a junior faculty member named Ebony, was supposed to speak instead. With little time left, Ebony shortened her presentation, which would be her first for a major institutional audience. Afterwards, during the reception, Ebony and John talk to a few of the hospital members who attended and ask questions about how the Centre was founded. Ebony starts to share the Centre's story, choosing her words carefully, when John steps in, 'I think what Ebony is trying to say is …' and proceeds to share his version and then concludes, 'You're doing great, kid; I'm behind you 100%'. In this situation, John took away valuable visibility time from someone they are saying they support, limiting Ebony's potential to make a name for herself across the institution and demonstrate her leadership skills. Additionally, John's attempt at 'supporting' Ebony during the conversation undermined her leadership position, attempting to 'save' her in this high-stakes conversation, further impacting her career potential in the eyes of the attendees. John talking more about his support of women than his quiet demonstration of that support is an example of performative 'saviour' allyship.

As we consider the continuum of allyship, we can also consider the continuum of change for those with dominant identities – and that these changes are not black and white, those with dominant identities are not either good or bad. The model of the Eight White Identities gives one example of a dominant identity and how no one is either a complete White abolitionist or White supremacist, but there is a continuum. No one is bad or good – everyone exists on a continuum that develops as they do (Box 12.6) [8].

Box 12.6 The Eight White Identities.

1 White Supremacist: clearly marked White society that preserves, names and values White supremacy.

2 White Voyeurism: wouldn't challenge a White supremacist; desires non-Whiteness because it's interesting, pleasurable; seeks to control the consumption and appropriation of non-Whiteness; fascination with culture (e.g. consuming Black culture without the burden of Blackness).

3 White Privilege: may critique supremacy but has a deep investment in questions of fairness/equality.

4 White Benefit: sympathetic to a set of issues but only privately; won't speak or act in solidarity publicly because they are benefiting through Whiteness in public (some people of colour [POC] are in this category as well).

5 White Confessional: some exposure to Whiteness takes place, but as a way of being accountable to POC after; seek validation from POC.

6 White Critical: take on board critiques of Whiteness and invest in exposing or marking the White regime; refuse to be complicit with the regime; Whiteness speaking back to Whiteness.

7 White Traitor: actively refuses complicity; names what's going on; the intention is to subvert White authority and tell the truth at whatever cost; needs them to dismantle institutions.

8 White Abolitionist: changing institutions, dismantling Whiteness and not allowing Whiteness to reassert itself.

Source: Hesse [8].

Intervening as an active bystander

What is bystander intervention/being an active bystander?

There are a few names for intervention frameworks used to interrupt biased, harassing, violent or other harmful behaviours. One framework that has grown in popularity recently is 'bystander intervention'. Bystander intervention is a behaviour tactic founded on de-escalation and anti-violence and was initially created to address street harassment. A critical element of this framework is that any intervention response must be focused on the target of the behaviour, not the bystander and their needs. This approach interrogates cultural and societal norms of behaviour to reset the status quo as one of support, care and anti-violence [9]. At its core, active bystander intervention is two things: first, recognising that a potentially harmful situation is about to occur or is occurring, and second, choosing to actively respond in a way that can positively influence the outcome.

How to recognise and intervene on the harm being witnessed

Often the first step to intervening is simply just to be able to recognise that harm is about to happen or has happened. We often call out harmful behaviour, and other witnesses didn't notice anything at all (Box 12.7).

Box 12.7 Recognising harm is the first step.

Go back to the case of Alice (Box 12.3) and the interrupting senior faculty member. Eric sticks around with the other faculty who seem to be holding back and chatting about something; he's curious about what they're talking about. Several faculty members console a Black female colleague, saying they're sorry she was treated that way during the meeting, and that it would never have happened to them as White faculty. Eric pulls one of the faculty aside and asks, 'What happened?'. The faculty member looks at him, a bit surprised: 'You didn't notice how awful he was to Renee? He kept interrupting her and wouldn't let her speak!' Eric is still confused: 'I think he's like that with everyone. I honestly didn't notice'. The faculty member rolls their eyes: 'He didn't do that to anyone else during the meeting'. Eric tries to remember if this was the case and why he didn't notice the interruption when others did.

Doing the personal self-reflection to understand when a harmful situation occurs takes intentional effort and open-mindedness, especially if someone explicitly tells you they were harmed. The '5 Ds of bystander intervention' is a common tactic described in intervention education (Box 12.8 and Box 12.9) [10].

Box 12.8 The 5Ds of bystander intervention.

Direct: do something yourself
- *Directly to the offender*: address the offender to interrupt the behaviour, using ally phrases (Box 12.9).
- *Directly to the target*: address the target to assess if they need or want help or if they would like to leave the situation.

Delegate: ask someone for help
If you are not in a position (physically or professionally) where you can safely interrupt the situation, delegate the intervention to someone else who can.

Distract: create a distraction
This will defuse or calm things down in the moment – this tactic should be used for emergencies with an imminent threat to safety or possible harm.

Delay: do something later
Similar to distraction, this should be used sparingly as the goal is to intervene in the moment. Depending on the circumstances, you may wait until after a situation or event to respond.

Document: record the incident
This is an increasingly effective tool of allyship to record situations of bias, harassment or other types of harm, so there is recorded evidence of the situation.

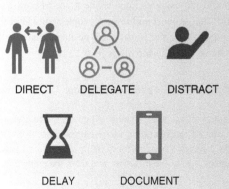

DIRECT   DELEGATE   DISTRACT

DELAY   DOCUMENT

Box 12.9 **Allyship phrases to use in the moment when harm occurs [9].**

- What did you mean by that?
- I'm surprised to hear that from you.
- Respond by stating what is important to you ('I don't believe in gay marriage' – 'I believe that all families deserve equality under the law').
- What makes you say/think that?
- I'm uncomfortable right now / I'm uncomfortable with that.
- I would like to understand that better. Help me understand your thinking.
- I didn't realise you thought that.
- Hold on; I need to process what you just said.
- What you just said is harmful.
- We don't say things like that here.
- Can you say that again?
- Ouch.

Reflection question
1 Think of a time you saw something biased / harassing / harmful occurring and didn't intervene. What was your barrier?
2 What would help you work through your barriers in the future?

Freedom to speak up

While training, frameworks and practice of allyship skills are some of the most important steps to establishing a culture of allyship, support from leadership and the organisation can be just as, if not more, important. Organisations interested in allyship must invest time and focus on what it means to create a culture of authentic accountability.

For allyship to truly make a difference in any environment, there must be a broad perception and practice that anyone in the organisation, regardless of level, can speak up, intervene and call someone 'in' or call someone 'out' on their harmful or biased behaviour. A person can call someone *out* for discriminatory behaviour by saying, 'Hey, that's not right', 'That language is racist' or 'What you said just then was sexist'. An ally can call *in* someone by saying, 'Ouch, that was really hurtful. Can I tell you why?', 'I'm surprised to hear that from you' or 'What did you mean when you said that?' Calling someone 'in', then, is a demonstration of what many in social justice circles call 'radical care or love'. By calling someone in that you know, there is a demonstration of care because you want to engage in a dialogue to understand each other so that the person can do better in the future.

Creating a culture of accountability requires hierarchical and dominant-oriented cultures like medicine and higher education to embrace all community members as part of the solution to bias, oppression and microaggressions. While it seems hard to imagine, organisations that support and reward people at any level for calling others 'in', especially senior leaders, will be able to harness the transformative change that allyship offers (Box 12.10).

Box 12.10 **Accountability starts at the top.**

A new medical school dean, an older White man, is holding his first town hall with all faculty and staff to get acquainted. At the end of his remarks, he says, 'I want to conclude by saying I am truly committed to diversity, equity and inclusion, and there are many things that

I don't know, so I am counting on you to hold me accountable and give me feedback if I step in it'. A few months later, he says something that many consider a microaggression but not overly offensive. You write him an email asking if you can give feedback and if he is open to it. The dean calls you and confirms he is open to feedback, after which you then have an open and honest conversation about his comments and how they made the group feel. He thanks you for the feedback and reconfirms that this is the type of information he wants to know about. A few months later, he uses an anonymised version of this story, admits he said something wrong, and publicly shares that he was thankful for the feedback, which was helpful. The next time you see your dean at a departmental get-together where the topic of DEI comes up, he offers some thoughts and mentions that you have been helpful in this area. In this scenario, not only was the dean authentically interested in feedback and welcoming when it was offered, but your career was not negatively impacted by offering this feedback through retaliation.

Embedding allyship and intervention in your organisation

One way to create a culture of accountability and embed support for being an active bystander in an organisation is by establishing community agreements. Community agreements are community-created norms and expectations that everyone agrees to use in the workplace environment. These agreements should be co-created by employees and leaders, provide ample time for community input and changes, and be created over time, as opposed to during a crisis or when a potentially heated situation is happening.

Some good examples of community agreements are from Alternate Roots [11] and Just Lead Washington [12]. These examples describe how your community, at various levels, all mutually agree to behave *and what actions the community and leaders take when an individual does not honour those agreements.*

The paradigm shifts at the individual level to begin authentic allyship also apply to institutions where organisations must move from 'some *need* support' to 'all *have* dignity, worth and a role to play in inclusion' (Table 12.3).

Advocacy and leadership driving accountability culture

There are two important things a leader can do for allyship. First, publicly and financially support programmes that expand allyship and create accountability across the organisation. 'Advocates and Allies' [13] is one example of an allyship group specifically for people who identify as men to have a safer space to get together and talk about their male allyship and explore questions together. Additionally, creating policies that establish a zero-tolerance approach to bias, harassment or other oppressive behaviours codifies actions that witnesses can take. Actively supporting these types of programmes as a leader is critical to creating spaces where allyship can develop.

Second, ensuring that those who speak out in the organisation against bias, harassment or other oppressive behaviours are not punished, either

Table 12.3 Institutional allyship perspective shift from some 'need' to all 'have'.

Some 'need'	All 'have'
A few identified targets	Everyone
Happens when problem arises	Implemented from day one
Mandatory for some	Mandatory for all
Closed, secret, stigmatised	Open, transparent, praised
Focus on remediation/response to failure	Focus on overall improvement/response to striving for excellence
Special accommodation	Usual provision

Just as Table 12.2 described the individual shift from 'me' to 'we', this table represents an institution's shift toward allyship in responding to harm. Institutions have traditionally addressed harm by handling remediation or situations one at a time and only when it needs addressing. In an institution that focuses on allyship, responding to and addressing harm is an institutional norm, is openly acknowledged and is implemented at the start of an employee's time at the institution. This paradigm shift is important for institutions to mitigate the historical stigma of harm and discrimination and instead encourage transparency and community support.

Source: Sunny Nakae, Sunshine Medical Education Consulting LLC©, 2019.

formally or informally. The buck stops with the leaders to ensure that those standing up against injustices aren't punished or face retaliation.

In any sector, it is essential to remember that what is rewarded socially and professionally will be reproduced. What is encouraged, in word and practice, becomes culture.

Further reading/resources

https://righttobe.org/guides/bystander-intervention-training (accessed 24 October 2022)

Guide to Allyship. https://guidetoallyship.com (accessed 25 October 2022)

Rothenberg, P.S. (2002) *White Privilege: Essential Readings on the Other Side of Racism*. New York: Worth Publishers.

Frey, W.R. (2020) White fragility: why it's so hard for white people to talk about racism. *Journal of Social Work*, **20** (1), 123–125.

Oluo, I. (2019) *So You Want to Talk about Race*. Seattle: Seal Press.

References

1 Bishop, A. (2015) *Becoming an Ally: Breaking the Cycle of Oppression in People*, 3e. Halifax: Fernwood Publishing.

2 Atcheson, S. Allyship – the key to unlocking the power of diversity Forbes. www.forbes.com/sites/shereeatcheson/2018/11/30/allyship-the-key-to-unlocking-the-power-of-diversity

3 Melaku, T., Beeman, A., Smith, D. and Johnson, W. (2020) Be a better ally. https://hbr.org/2020/11/be-a-better-ally%C2%A0

4 Fosberg, A., Bynum, A. and Tripp, H. (2021) How do you distinguish effective allyship from performative allyship? https://pennstatelaw.psu.edu/news/effective-allyship-part-one

5 Indigenous Action (2014) Accomplices not allies: abolishing the ally industrial complex. www.indigenousaction.org/accomplices-not-allies-abolishing-the-ally-industrial-complex

6 Edwards, K.E. (2006) Aspiring social justice ally identity development: a conceptual model. *NASPA Journal*, **43** (4), 39–60.

7 Taylor, S. (n.d.) The body is not an apology. www.sonyareneetaylor.com/the-body-is-not-an-apology

8 Hesse, B. (n.d.) The 8 White Identities, by Barnor Hesse. Breaking down the white gaze. https://reverseracism.tumblr.com/post/57939811587/the-8-white-identities-by-barnor-hesse-breaking

9 Katz, J. (2018) Bystander training as leadership training: notes on the origins, philosophy, and pedagogy of the mentors in violence prevention model. *Violence Against Women*, **24** (15), 1755–1776.

10 Right to Be (n.d.) The 5Ds of bystander intervention. https://righttobe.org/guides/bystander-intervention-training.

11 Alternate Roots (2018) Alternate Roots Community Agreements. https://alternateroots.org/alternate-roots-community-agreements.

12 Just Lead Washington (n.d.) REJI organizational toolkit & guides. https://justleadwa.org/learn/rejitoolkit

13 North Dakota State University (n.d.) Advocates and Allies Project. www.ndsu.edu/forward/projects/advocate_forward/advocates_and_allies_project

CHAPTER 13

Teaching Equality, Diversity and Inclusion in Healthcare

Sylk Sotto-Santiago

Indiana University School of Medicine, Indianapolis, IN, USA

OVERVIEW

- Medical education plays a critical role as a key lever for addressing health disparities.
- Teaching and incorporating equality, diversity and inclusion into the curriculum recognises that all concepts are interconnected.
- To create inclusive learning environments, educators and leaders must engage diversity as a collective resource, create opportunities for sharing a multiplicity of identities, and offer connections between the lesson and societal needs.
- Multiple frameworks offer a curricular structure for teaching equality, diversity and inclusion: structural competence and cultural humility; antiracist education, decolonisation and critical race theory.

Introduction

Today's medical education spans a rich continuum of undergraduate and postgraduate training with continuing professional education. Its goal is to provide society with the most knowledgeable and skilled healthcare workforce. The call to teach equality, diversity and inclusion (EDI) in healthcare represents a necessary change. We need to teach EDI to address health disparities with the collective goal of health equity. Health disparities negatively affect groups of people that have systematically experienced greater social or economic obstacles to health. These obstacles stem from characteristics historically linked to discrimination or exclusion, such as race or ethnicity, religion, socioeconomic status, gender, mental health, sexual orientation or geographic location. We can achieve health equity if we are guided by medical education and academic medicine's social mission. Defining concepts and terms specific to medical education and frameworks to guide the curricular design is essential to achieving this goal.

Equitable patient-centred care

To achieve our goal, medical professionals need to move towards *equitable patient-centred care* which takes into consideration the specific needs of the patient. It does not vary in quality based on personal characteristics like gender, ethnicity, geographic location, religion,

sexuality, socioeconomic status, etc. Equitable patient-centred care reflects the need for a healthcare workforce that demonstrates structural competency (Box 13.1) [1].

Box 13.1 **Structural competency.**

Structural competency is the ability to discern how issues defined clinically as symptoms, attitudes or diseases also represent matters of food and safe water access, urban and rural infrastructures or definitions of illness and wellbeing, to name a few [2]. Structural competency incorporates multidisciplinary fields into medical education and clinical training. It prepares the healthcare workforce to recognise, act and connect history and current sociopolitical environments with the effects on health equity within the population, often along social categories. [2]

Equitable patient-centred care and structural competency require individuals in the healthcare workforce to address their implicit and explicit biases and reflect on the impact of these biases on the care they provide [2]. Where can we provide these opportunities? During medical education and clinical training. Without question, our healthcare systems and society need serious reforms.

The consequences of historical inaction have been growing health disparities that ultimately have a substantial adverse impact on the same systems and society. Medical education plays a critical role as a key lever for change and establishing professional standards that inform medical practice [3]. Teaching and incorporating EDI into the curriculum recognise that all concepts are interconnected in ways that make the goal clear: health equity.

As we consider medical education and academic medicine, we must consider the reclamation of this mission toward health equity (Box 13.2).

Box 13.2 **Health equity.**

According to the World Health Organization, *health equity* is the absence of unfair, avoidable or irremediable differences among people, whether those groups are defined socially, economically, demographically, geographically or by other dimensions of inequality.

> Social factors and norms shape the distribution of power and the availability and distribution of health resources.
>
> Source: World Health Organization (n.d.) Health Equity. www.who. int/health-topics/health-equity.

Medical education needs to be guided by the mission of improving the health of the public and the obligation to facilitate and support a broader social responsibility [4,5]. Academic medicine is a critical part of the discovery and development of fundamental principles, effective health policies and best practices that advance research and education in the health sciences, ultimately to improve the health and wellbeing of individuals and populations [5].

Defining equality, diversity and inclusion in medical education

Diversity embodies all aspects of human differences. It serves as a catalyst for change, resulting in equality, equal opportunities, access, care and outcomes. The exercise of intentional inclusion is critical for successfully achieving diversity. Inclusion is achieved by nurturing the climate and culture of the institution through the active inclusion of its diverse members. The objective is to create an environment that fosters a sense of belonging and respect and recognises everyone's values. This action is increasingly understood as non-negotiable and of extreme importance in preparing an innovative and representative workforce, addressing health disparities and inequities, advancing science and serving the needs of the public and society [6].

To create inclusive learning environments, educators and leaders in educational institutions must engage diversity as a collective resource, create opportunities for sharing a multiplicity of intersecting identities, and offer connections between the lesson and societal needs [6].

I want to offer two additional concepts: equity and a sense of belonging. Not all work and learning environments are created equally. To be an institution that truly embraces the values of EDI, *equity* is needed. Equity recognises that we do not all start from the same place; societal systems must acknowledge and adjust imbalances. Through equity, organisations provide the required resources for all individuals to reach shared and equal goals. Second, *belonging* is the experience of being accepted, included and valued. A fundamental human motivation, a sense of belonging positively influences an individual's health, abilities, relationships and overall wellbeing [7]. Encountering racism, discrimination, bias, microaggressions and covert exclusionary practices interferes with the experience of belonging in educational environments and the learning process. A lack of belonging contributes to isolation and further marginalisation, mistrust, emotional distress, lessened effectiveness, exhaustion and taxation, and possibly serious health issues [7].

Teaching EDI in healthcare focuses on ensuring that learners gain knowledge, skills and attitudes consistent with a view of patients as complex individuals, representing themselves and not entire cultures. Medical education should prepare the healthcare workforce to recognise, act and connect history and current sociopolitical environments with the impact on health equity.

The art of inclusive teaching in medical education

Paulo Freire's early conception of humanisation in education encouraged educators to listen to learners and build knowledge and experiences that help educators engage in a dynamic and personalised education approach with the goal of social transformation [8]. Teaching EDI is a critical part of that transformation. Inclusive teaching offers a model for the exploration of lived experiences as educators, but also those of our learners. Inclusive teaching also includes inclusive pedagogies and culturally relevant teaching practices (Figure 13.1) [9].

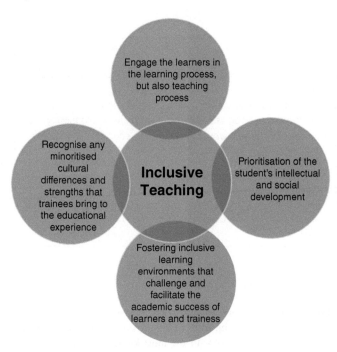

Figure 13.1 Inclusive teaching.
Source: Adapted from Danowitz and Tuitt [9].

There are several strategies which can be incorporated into an inclusive teaching curriculum (Table 13.1).

Adopting these strategies fosters equitable environments in which learners feel welcomed and have a sense of belonging, and the instructors can utilise them to combat inequities in the system [9]. Educators can work towards inclusive teaching by assessing learners' prior knowledge, planning lessons that account for those differences, and incorporating teaching practices that encourage equal participation from all learners (Box 13.3).

> Box 13.3 **Mispronouncing a student's name.**
>
> Dr Mistry is happy to have a medical student do a clinical rotation with him. He is unsure how to pronounce the student's name, Oghenekevwe Okoh, and is uncertain if this will cause any upset or offence. When introducing Oghenekevwe to the rest of the team on the first day, he instead refers to him as 'the medical student'. When they return to his room, Dr Mistry asks Oghenekevwe how to pronounce his name. Oghenekevwe explains the pronunciation several times, but Dr Mistry laughs and says, 'That's too much of a mouthful. Can I call you Oggi instead?'.

Table 13.1 Strategies for inclusive teaching.

Strategy	Action	Reason
1. Incorporate diverse perspectives	Expand reading material to include diverse authors and/or offer diverse examples in case studies	Case studies offer an opportunity to break stereotypes. Does the case study describe patients in obsolete gendered roles?
2. Create and sustain inclusive learning environments	Encourage all learners to participate and engage in conversation. Establish ground rules for controversial topics or those that discuss deeper societal contexts	Maintain high expectations for yourself as educator and facilitator of the learning process. Expect the same awareness and engagement from your students
3. Supportive structures	Be flexible with additional learning support	Are your office hours of mentoring and advice at times difficult for students to attend?
4. Examine unconscious biases	Reflect on your own attitudes towards students. Who are you mentoring? Who are you not mentoring? Why?	Request peer review of your teaching and ask the evaluator to specifically observe who you are calling on to participate. Are there differences in your grading patterns?
5. Request student feedback	Do not wait until the end of the course to request feedback. Do it periodically	Continuing to monitor and adjust based on learning goals. This type of check-in also helps educators understand the learning environment and climate
6. Co-create content	Have you considered that students can contribute to diverse case studies and are able to see society from a different generational lens?	Co-creation is important in learning engagement, but it also raises awareness for the educator. Learners share new knowledge and bring awareness of issues, and it opens communication for expressing concerns and opportunities

Oghenekevwe feels very upset at his name being laughed at. His Nigerian background places great emphasis on the name given to a child, and he feels disrespected by how his supervisor has not taken the time or effort to learn his name.

Due to Oghenekevwe's fear of causing his supervisor to be upset with him or not passing him on his clinical attachment, Oghenekevwe agrees to be called 'Oggi' despite the distress that it causes him. Oghenekevwe then starts introducing himself as 'Oggi' at future placements to avoid having his name laughed at again.

Simple techniques that ensure a welcoming, inclusive environment for all learners include properly pronouncing students' names. Making an effort to pronounce their name correctly demonstrates respect and honours the individual, their history and the meaning of their name.

Faculty educational and instructional development programmes are needed to develop excellence in medical education. These programmes are not consistently established across institutions, and clinician educators have often delivered teaching in a manner that speaks to their personal values, learning modalities and role modelling from their educational journeys. Clinical and administrative duties can be a barrier to these educators engaging in their own personal and professional development in medical education. Inclusive teaching is still a critical requirement to advance health equity, whether the onus is on the individual educator or (more likely) the institution. This is an art to be nurtured.

Extant literature demonstrates trends in curricular design in medical education, inclusive of eight broad categories: cross-cultural exchanges, early clinical and community experience, e-learning, interprofessional education (IPE), portfolios, problem-based learning (PBL), scholarly concentrations (SCs) and self-directed learning (SDL) (Table 13.2) [10,11].

Frameworks for incorporating equality, diversity and inclusion in healthcare

The foundation for inclusive teaching and inclusive learning environments in medical education must acknowledge the ontology of history, challenging the relationship between medical knowledge and lived experiences of minoritised populations [9]. To better apply inclusive teaching practices, we need to think about frameworks that may offer an overarching structure.

Equality, diversity and inclusion and related concepts embedded in curricula are limited, often just superficial and not thoroughly integrated. The following frameworks may offer an overarching structure from which to draw inclusive teaching practices.

- Structural competence and cultural humility.
- Antiracist education, decolonisation and critical race theory.

Structural competence and cultural humility

Throughout the years, cultural competence had to evolve from making assumptions about patients based on their background to implementing the principles of patient-centred care, including exploration, empathy and responsiveness to patients' needs, values and preferences. However, it also developed into the assumption that the healthcare workforce would become competent in specific cultures as if there was an endpoint. This approach gave rise to generalisations of groups and solidified negative stereotypes. The same culturally competent providers must expand their skill sets to include skills instrumental in cross-cultural interactions. These cross-cultural interactions must be considered in the context of the core competencies outlined by the Liaison Committee on Medical Education (LCME) and the General Medical Council (GMC). They accredit medical schools in the USA/Canada and the UK respectively (Box 13.4).

Box 13.4 **Core competencies.**

You may ask: Do all physicians need to understand the role of race/ethnicity and gender in thinking about the patient and their pharmacology and disease?

Fact: Current literature emphasises the importance of cultural competence in engaging the diversity of patients and associated health outcomes.

In 2022, the GMC undertook a stakeholder and public consultation regarding amendments to the revised Good Medical Practice (GMP) guidelines. It is hoped that the next iteration of the GMP will

Table 13.2 Curricular design in medical education.

Cross-cultural exchanges	Educational and training experiences within diverse communities promote cultural humility and structural competence. Learners will develop an increased awareness of resource allocation, empathy, equitable patient-centred professional practice and significant public health issues. Scholars have found that learners valued the learning experience and broadened their perspectives while facilitation increased confidence, independence and realistic goal-setting ability
Early clinical and community experience	Early clinical and community experience relates to cross-cultural exchanges and appears to strengthen and contextualise learning
Innovative teaching modalities	Innovative teaching modalities, such as e-learning, can enhance accessibility in ways that serve learning differences
Interprofessional education	Interprofessional education offers more professional opportunities to learn about, from and with each other towards effective collaboration and improving health outcomes
Problem-based learning	Problem-based learning is a common pedagogical approach that aims to facilitate student learning by immersing students in healthcare practice problems. Problem-based learning in medical education is relied on heavily as it increases the depth of learners' knowledge and helps them retain facts for extended periods, a critical part of clinical training
Scholarly concentrations	By incorporating scholarly concentrations exploring EDI and fundamental structural and social determinants of health discussion, medical education may introduce differential medical practices dependent on where healthcare systems might be situated
Self-directed learning	By incorporating self-directed learning, educators offer reflective inquiry and active learning opportunities

Source: Adapted from Onyura et al. [11].

incorporate the expectation that clinicians will be aware of health inequalities and their impact on the patient care being provided.

Source: www.gmc-uk.org/ethical-guidance/good-medical-practice-review

Structural competence

We know that health disparities are caused by social and structural determinants of health (SSDH). SSDH refers to the complex, integrated and overlapping social structures and economic systems responsible for most health inequities (see also Chapters 2 and 4). These social structures and economic systems include the social environment, physical environment, health services and structural and societal factors. Social determinants of health are shaped by the distribution of money, power and resources throughout local communities, nations and the world. Yet, medical education often perpetuates biological and cultural notions of racial and ethnic health disparities.

Structural competence is defined by how healthcare systems reflect racially diverse patients in terms of pathogenisation, hospitalisation and resulting life chances [2]. Moreover, by teaching structural competence, medical education helps examine how the healthcare workforce and providers have traditionally learned about race and racism and how institutions or healthcare systems mobilise to connect health and wealth inequalities [2]. By embedding EDI in medical education and utilising structural competence as a framework, educators would recognise structures that shape clinical interactions, rearticulate cultural formulations in structural terms, observe or enact structural interventions and develop humility. This notion of structural humility, where healthcare providers collaborate across disciplines with community members, is a challenging process [2]. Its predecessor, cultural humility, is even more relevant today [12] (Box 13.5).

Box 13.5 **Teaching the importance of cultural competency.**

Dr Mersha believes in the impact of structural and social determinants of health, such as housing, food access, transportation, etc., on health outcomes. He has learned more about equality, equity, diversity, inclusion and accessibility. He wants to demonstrate the concept of structural competence with his students. However, he is concerned that this would require a change in his curriculum.

Understanding the importance of teaching structural competency, Dr Mersha incorporates a specific five-minute section at the end of his case-based discussions with students, asking them to consider what structural and social determinants of health were specific to the case that has been discussed.

Medical education needs healthcare professionals to think about how such variables as race, class, gender and ethnicity are shaped by both the interactions of individuals in the exam room and the learning environment. Simple techniques include discussions during debriefing of a patient and discussing the larger structural contexts in which their interactions occur. Journal clubs, rounds, morbidity and mortality conferences, etc. provide a space in which to discuss: What else affected the outcome of this case? What structural and/or social determinants of health were at play?

Whichever method you use to teach structural competence, it does not require an overhaul of teaching sessions but can include simple steps to introduce the concepts for the students to consider on a frequent basis.

Cultural humility

Cultural humility is a life-long process of self-reflection and self-critique with the goal of recognising the inherent power in the healthcare provider–patient relationship [12]. Cultural humility requires healthcare providers to engage in conversations with patients, communities, colleagues and themselves. It is crucial for healthcare providers first to acknowledge the set of assumptions and beliefs determined by an individual's upbringing and growth. Furthermore, cultural humility emphasises actively listening to patients to counter the power inequities in the clinical encounter, delivering a high-quality patient experience.

Applying cultural humility helps to avoid stereotyping, making healthcare providers also learners with curiosity about patient beliefs, thus fostering mutually respectful partnerships with patients and communities. The most important lesson is that cultural humility does not have an endpoint, as cultural competence suggests, but being in a relationship that evolves [12].

Cultural humility is crucial to training global healthcare professionals. It should be at the centre of the healthcare curriculum to allow learners to be educated in EDI principles, approaches and skills that contribute to respectful and productive patient relationships. Healthcare providers who embrace EDI and cultural humility consistently consider patients' beliefs and learn to appreciate culture in its broadest sense and dynamic state (Box 13.6).

Box 13.6 Reflective exercise.

Cultural humility begins with ourselves. Embracing cultural humility requires introspection.
Consider the following reflection questions.

1 What tools can you use for reflection? Journalling, sharing about your life with others?
2 Think about the pivotal moments of your life that shaped who you are today.
3 Privilege comes in many forms. Have you considered the opportunities and challenges along your own professional journey?
4 What about the encounter with your patient? Did you demonstrate empathy? Did any bias you may hold play a role in a conversation with a patient or a colleague?

Antiracist education, decolonisation and critical race theory

Antiracist education

Antiracist education emerged from the broader field of multicultural education to dismantle racism through developing new curricula and positive pedagogic practices [13]. Antiracist education creates inclusive learning environments that engage and acknowledge the discomfort, tensions and vulnerability when addressing issues centred on race. It serves as a tool to transform medical education with knowledge and skills, empowering educators and learners through teaching, agency and activism. Similarly, when teaching EDI in healthcare, antiracist education counters the history, structure and culture of racism (Box 13.7) [13].

Decolonisation

While it may take some time for the concept of decolonisation to be embraced in medical education, scholars and practitioners should also focus on systems transformation, which is critical for EDI efforts. Systems and practices that do not attempt to disrupt the dominant systems serve as hindrances to health justice and equity. In the case of academic medicine, historically underrepresented faculty and learners are often isolated and marginalised. Without decentring dominance, we leave the same structures in place and become complicit in the

---

Box 13.7 Antiracist education.

Phases of antiracist medical education

Foundational awareness	Example: An institution or organisation may mandate explicit training, such as implicit bias Example: Unequivocal messaging by the leadership to raise awareness and set institutional direction in high visibility venues
Foundational knowledge	Example: Knowledge goes beyond awareness by developing more intentional and intensive programmes such as courses specifically discussing race in medicine or SSDH and its significance in the communities we serve. It is important to discuss and debate the structures in place that led to the current state
Embedding practices	Example: Students can provide curricular feedback by participating in the review of curricular elements and examples that reinforce biases and racism
Dismantling phase	Example: University admissions and student affairs leadership can identify and dismantle systemic racism in the admissions process, such as reviewing admission criteria that impact equal access and prevent student success

Antiracist education starts with foundational awareness, progressively advances through foundational knowledge, embedding an antiracist lens into related practices, and contributes to dismantling oppressive structures.

Source: Adapted from Sotto-Santiago et al. [13].

---

status quo, a status quo full of inequality. Decolonisation suggests challenging institutionalised power and privilege; undoing historical hierarchies of power, knowledge and otherness; and being taught to navigate our world and understand what is legitimate through the eyes and words of the colonised [14].

Critical race theory

Critical race theory (CRT) (Box 13.8) also holds potential for the field of medical education. Guided by CRT tenets, we can incorporate racialised perspectives into academia throughout curriculum, administration and EDI initiatives [15]. This opportunity will bring awareness about the role of institutions in producing and perpetuating health disparities and recognise the systemic complexities that further disadvantage marginalised groups in society.

Box 13.8 Critical race theory.

Critical race theory interrogates the role of race and racism in society and how they have impacted policy and practices at all levels. Emerging from legal scholars in the US, it critiques how the social construction of race perpetuates a system that relegates people of colour to the bottom tiers. CRT also recognises that race intersects with other identities, including ethnicity, gender and sexuality, among others internalised by individuals [15].

Incorporating CRT into the foundation of medical education and transforming curriculum development, among other institutional functions, may be an essential step in our work to train and educate the next generation of healthcare providers and build a better, more just society.

Moving forward

Teaching EDI in healthcare requires teaching against oppression and inequity. EDI curricular development shares common threads of self-reflection in identity, power and positionality. It requires us to 'unlearn and relearn' truths about history's relationship with race, leading to health disparities. Clinician educators must move to elevate equitable patient-centred care and embed culturally aware and socially responsible curricula as an inclusive teaching model in medical education.

Enacting inclusive teaching in medical education

Recently, we explored the integration of EDI content into medical education as not an end unto itself but part of a more significant effort to improve the ability of the healthcare workforce in their roles as equity-minded practitioners and healthcare advocates [16]. Healthcare provider preparedness is predicated upon exposure to, immersion in and critical reflection on the appropriate foundational knowledge, skills, dispositions and experiences to approach clinical practice, medical science and healing in ways that affirm the worth and preserve the dignity of individuals, families and communities. The integration of EDI in curricular development is designed to equip future healthcare providers to enter their careers as lifelong learners with the agency, awareness and capacity to act as agents of change with patients, families, other health professionals and policymakers to:

- improve equity, access and quality of care to patients and families from increasingly diverse and unequally resourced communities
- contribute to and enhance team-based clinical and community-based care
- engage in advocacy and practice that improve policy and strengthen health and healthcare systems.

We proposed nine domains to embed EDI with the medical education curriculum: disparities and factors influencing health; community engagement; bias, stigma and stereotyping in professional practice; intercultural communication; use of interpreters; self-awareness, cultural humility and reflexivity; patient and family engagement; negotiating intersectionality in professional practice; and physician orientation to and role in healthcare advocacy (Box 13.9). These domains can be used to help ensure that students gain needed knowledge, skills and attitudes consistent with healthcare providers' oath to patients, but also the values of EDI.

Box 13.9 **Incorporating EDI into the medical education curriculum.**

Domain	Proposed curriculum for Culturally Aware and Socially Responsible Medical Education
Disparities and factors influencing health	Describe the social determinants of health and their influences on patient and population outcomes
Community engagement	Community engagement is the application of institutional resources to address and solve health challenges facing communities through collaboration with these communities. It often involves partnerships and coalitions that help mobilise resources, influence political and health systems and serve as catalysts for changing policies, programmes and practices
Bias, stigma and stereotyping	Bias, stigma and stereotyping incorporate mental associations that take place without intention, awareness or control, challenge undesirable stereotypes and fight prejudice
Intercultural communication	Intercultural communication is the verbal and non-verbal exchange of information between and among people from different cultural backgrounds. A large body of scholarship focuses on people's interface with different cultures and the influence of cultural backgrounds and identities on one's worldview
Use of interpreters	Skilled communication is needed to serve the needs of a patient population with limited language proficiency
Self-awareness, cultural humility and reflexivity	Cultural humility and reflexivity underscore the lifelong commitment to learning that the healthcare workforce makes but also involves self-evaluation, self-critiquing and redressing power imbalances. Reflexivity exercises expand the ability to understand how one's social locations and experiences of advantage or disadvantage have shaped how one understands the world
Physician orientation to and role in healthcare advocacy	A healthcare provider's role in health advocacy promotes those social, economic, educational and political changes that ameliorate the suffering and threats to human health and wellbeing they identify through their professional work and expertise
Negotiating intersectionality in professional practice	Recognise the implications of intersectionality. Recognise how different or combinations of identities impact the healthcare team's attitudes

| Patient and family engagement | Patient and family engagement is a method for planning, delivering and evaluating healthcare grounded in principles of mutually beneficial partnerships among patients, families and healthcare professionals. This approach implements the core concepts of trust, respect, dignity, communication and collaboration within these relationships |

Source: Adapted from Price et al. [16].

Conclusion

The dismantling of systemic barriers that perpetuate health disparities begins with an honest reflection on the role of healthcare providers and educators. However, the state of instructional and educational development in this area is limited, especially when it requires teaching against oppression and inequity. The success of EDI curricula in healthcare relies on devoted and excellent teachers, believers in the importance of EDI and allies in the fight for equality, and robust infrastructure and resources with an explicit, high-quality education that engages learners.

By understanding and adopting the frameworks outlined in this chapter, educational institutions can ensure that healthcare learners gain much needed knowledge, skills and attitudes consistent with equitable patient-centred care.

Reflection

As an academic, I hope that academic medicine centres produce a healthcare workforce that fights to eradicate health disparities and works towards health equity, embracing inclusive teaching practices under several of the frameworks discussed, but especially for me, cultural humility.

My philosophy as an educator is to be an equity-centred teacher who creates an inclusive and supportive learning environment; a genuine and authentic partner in instruction who is still curious about learning; and a teacher who 'conspires' to think critically about the more significant roles of institutions and identity in health and education.

References

1 Maldonado, M., Dupras, D. and Sotto-Santiago, S. (2019) Moving Beyond Cultural Competence Toward Cultural Humility and the Delivery of Equitable Patient-Centered Care. https://scholarworks.iupui.edu/bitstream/handle/1805/29375/Moving%20Beyond%20Cultural%20Competence%20Toward%20Equitable%20Patient%20Centered%20Communication%2019.pdf?sequence=1&isAllowed=y

2 Metzl, J. and Hansen, H. (2014) Structural competency: theorizing a new medical engagement with stigma and inequality. *Social Science and Medicine*, **103**, 126–133.

3 Smith, D.G. (2012) Building institutional capacity for diversity and inclusion in academic medicine. *Academic Medicine*, **87** (11), 1511–1515.

4 Ramsey, P.G. and Miller, E.D. (2009) A single mission for academic medicine: improving health. *JAMA*, **301** (14), 1475–1476.

5 Sotto-Santiago, S., Sharp, S., Mac, J. et al. (2021) Reclaiming the mission of academic medicine: an examination of institutional responses to (anti) racism. *AEM Education and Training*, **5**: S33–S43.

6 Roberts, L. (2020) Belonging, respectful inclusion, and diversity in medical education. *Academic Medicine*, **95** (5), 661–664.

7 Tuitt, F. et al. (2016) *Race, Equity, and the Learning Environment: The Global Relevance of Critical and Inclusive Pedagogies in Higher Education*. Sterling: Stylus Publishing.

8 Freire, P. (2021) *Pedagogy of Hope: Reliving Pedagogy of the Oppressed*. London: Bloomsbury Publishing.

9 Danowitz, M.A. and Tuitt, F.A. (2010) Moving towards inclusive excellence in doctoral studies. In: *Making Inclusion Work: Experiences from Academia Around the World* (eds S. Katila, S. Meriläinen and J. Tienari), 33–47. Cheltenham: Edward Elgar.

10 Addy, T.M., Hafler, J. and Galerneau, F. (2016) Faculty development for fostering clinical reasoning skills in early medical students using a modified Bayesian approach. *Teaching and Learning in Medicine*, **28** (4), 415–423.

11 Onyura, B., Baker, L., Cameron, B. et al. (2016) Evidence for curricular and instructional design approaches in undergraduate medical education: an umbrella review. *Medical Teacher*, **38** (2), 150–161.

12 Tervalon, M. and Murray-Garcia, J. (1998) Cultural humility versus cultural competence: a critical distinction in defining physician training outcomes in multicultural education. *Journal of Health Care for the Poor and Underserved*, **9** (2), 117–125.

13 Sotto-Santiago, S., Poll-Hunter, N., Trice, T. et al. (2021) A framework for developing antiracist medical educators and practitioner-scholars. *Academic Medicine*, **97** (1), 41–47.

14 Tuck, E., McKenzie, M. and McCoy, K. (2014) Land education: indigenous, post-colonial, and decolonizing perspectives on place and environmental education research. *Environmental Education Research*, **20** (1), 1–23.

15 Stefancic, J. and Delgado, R. (1995) *Critical Race Theory: The Cutting Edge*. Philadelphia: Temple University Press.

16 Price, M., Sotto-Santiago, S., Lazarus, K. and Christy, L. (2018) Culturally Appropriate & Socially Responsive Care [CASRC] thread. https://scholarworks.iupui.edu/bitstream/handle/1805/29376/Culturally%20Appropriate%20and%20Socially%20Responsive%20Care%20Final%202018.pdf?sequence=2&isAllowed=y

Index

ABC of Equality, Diversity and Inclusion in Healthcare, First Edition. Edited by Shehla Imtiaz-Umer and John Frain.
© 2023 John Wiley & Sons Ltd. Published 2023 by John Wiley & Sons Ltd.